Curing Arthritis Naturally

with Chinese Medicine

Douglas Frank & Bob Flaws

BLUE POPPY PRESS

For my Mother and Father

Douglas Frank

Published by:

BLUE POPPY PRESS, INC.
1775 LINDEN AVE.
BOULDER, CO 80304

First Edition, November, 1997

ISBN 0-936185-87-2
LC 97-71728

COMP Designation: Original work using a standard translational
terminology

Printed at Johnson's Printing in Boulder, CO
on essentially chlorine-free paper
Cover design by Jeff Fuller of Crescent Moon

10 9 8 7 6 5 4 3 2 1

Table of Contents

Introduction

Between 35 and 40 million Americans are affected by arthritis. It is one of the most prevalent chronic health problems in the United States with a cost of $64.8 billion per year in medical care and lost wages.[1] Among those 65 years and older, arthritis is epidemic with an estimated 65-85% of all Americans in this age group suffering from joint pain ranging in severity from a minor inconvenience to a severely disabling disease. Even people under 45 may suffer from arthritis as the result of traumatic injury and/or surgery.

What is arthritis?

Arthritis means joint (*arthr-*) inflammation (*-itis*). When prefaced by the word osteo, it simply means inflammation of the joints of the bones. Other names for osteoarthritis (OA) are degenerative joint disease (DJD), osteoarthroses (*i.e.*, bone joint condition), and hypertrophic osteoarthritis. It is the most common of all forms of joint disease, typically first appearing asymptomatically in the 20s and 30s and becoming universal by age 70. As the authors of *The Merck Manual*, one of the "bibles" of Western MDs, says, "Almost all persons by age 40 have some pathologic changes in the weight-bearing joints, although relatively few people are symptomatic [by that age]."[2]

---

[1] "Arthritis Fact Sheet," Arthritis Foundation, Atlanta, GA, p. 1, May, 1997

[2] *The Merck Manual of Diagnosis & Therapy*, 15th edition, ed. by Robert Berkow, Merck Sharp & Dohme Research Laboratories, Rahway, NJ, 1987, p. 1258)

Rheumatoid arthritis (RA) is by far the most serious, painful, and potentially crippling form of arthritis. It is a chronic systemic disease characterized by flare-ups and remissions. RA affects two million people in the United States, mostly women. Rheumatoid arthritis attacks the joints primarily but may affect the supporting connective tissues throughout the body, causing fever, weakness, fatigue, and deformity. The cause of RA is not known, but a hereditary predisposition and an environmental agent, such as a virus, are suspected.[3]

Do men and women both suffer from arthritis equally?

While both men and women get arthritis, the incidence in women is significantly higher—about two to one. However, its onset is typically earlier in men than in women. Osteoarthritis is found in all climates throughout the world. In fact, OA occurs in almost all vertebrates. The only two mammals it does not occur in are bats and sloths which both spend much of their lives hanging upside down!

What causes arthritis?

According to modern Western medicine, its etiology or cause is unknown. OA appears to be due to a complex set of interacting mechanical, biological, biochemical, and enzymatic feedback loops. When one or more of these components fails to do its job properly, this sets in motion the changes in the tissue of the joints we call arthritis. Some of the factors which may contribute to the onset of arthritis are congenital joint abnormalities, genetic defects, infectious, metabolic, endocrine, and neuropathic diseases, virtually any disease which alters the normal structure and function of the cartilage covering the inner surfaces of the joint, and acute and chronic trauma affecting this cartilage. In terms of this last cause, we are talking about wear and tear. Any motion which

---

[3] "Arthritis," Microsoft (R) Encarta, 1994, Funk & Wagnalls Corporation

repeatedly puts stress on the inner surfaces of the joint may result in micro-trauma leading eventually to inflammation. When this kind of micro-trauma continues year after year, as in certain occupations such as foundry workers and bus drivers, a whole series of micro-trauma sooner or later adds up to significant damage to the surfaces of the joints. Whether this happens sooner or later often depends on other factors affecting our health, such as our metabolism, our hormones, our immune system, and various infectious diseases.

What are the signs and symptoms of arthritis?

The onset of arthritis is usually subtle and gradual and begins by affecting only one or two joints. Its first symptom is pain and this pain is typically made worse by exercise. When one wakes up in the morning, the affected joint may be stiff, but this improves with movement after 15-30 minutes. As the disease progresses, joint mobility becomes diminished and flexion contractures occur. One may hear a grating noise and feel a grating sensation within the joint when it is moved. This is called crepitus. Eventually, the affected joints become enlarged and may even become hot to the touch and red in color. As the ligaments holding the joint in place become lax, the joint may become increasingly unstable and increasingly painful. Tenderness on palpation around the affected joint and pain on passive motion (*i.e.*, when someone else moves the joint for you) are late signs in the progression of this disease. Adding insult to injury, muscular spasms add to the pain. Eventually, as the inflammatory process continues to affect the cartilage and underlying bone tissue, the joint may become deformed, the surrounding muscles may atrophy, and nodular pseudocysts may appear.

How does Western medicine diagnosis arthritis?

The Western medical diagnosis of arthritis is usually based on the above signs and symptoms. When there are no signs and symptoms, sometimes a diagnosis is made through x-ray. If

3

arthritis is due to gout or rheumatoid arthritis (RA), both systemic diseases, blood sedimentation rates may help confirm this. Otherwise blood sedimentation rates are normal or are only slightly elevated.[4]

How does Western medicine treat arthritis?

The main treatment of arthritis by Western medicine is through the use of over-the-counter and prescription nonsteroidal anti-inflammatory's (NSAIDs). There are over 20 of these in common use in the United States, including aspirin, Tylenol, Advil, Motrin, Naprosyn, Alleve, Orudis, and Feldene. However, according to Dr. Jason Theodosakis,

> What's curious is that while these drug companies come out with new versions of the same thing, an anti-inflammatory agent, osteoarthritis is mostly non-inflammatory. Only occasionally do you find inflammation in the later stages of the disease. Furthermore, there is some preliminary evidence that when you put anti-inflammatory pills in a culture with cartilage cells, it impairs the healing process. So you're covering up the pain but probably impairing the healing process and stopping the signals that you have joint pain... they do not address the cause of the disease and may in fact worsen it.[5]

One of the effects of NSAIDs and aspirin usage not commonly mentioned in the medical literature, such as *The Merck Manual*, is that they impair cartilage repair. In fact, NSAIDs and aspirin usage has been linked to *increased cartilage destruction!*[5] This side effect is ironic since most users of NSAIDs and aspirin are people with osteoarthritis caused by cartilage damage in the first

---

[4] Eosinophil sedimentation rates (ESR) are an indication of infection and inflammation.

[5] Theodosakis, Jason, "The Amazing Cure for Arthritis: An interview with Jason Theodosakis, M.D., M.S., M.H.P.", *Nexus, Colorado's Holistic Journal*, Boulder, CO, May/June 1997, p. 27

place. Dr. Theodosakis goes on to say that, "When you give people anti-inflammatory pills, even in the highest doses, only 70 percent get pain relief."[6]

Unfortunately, the use of NSAIDs also often has side effects. The most common side effect is gastrointestinal irritation and ulceration. One study found that 1/3 of bleeding ulcers in seniors over 60 years of age is due to aspirin and NSAIDs.[2] The long-term use of acetaminophen and NSAIDs are controversial even within Western medicine. Research has found that taking more than 1,000 acetaminophen pills, such as Tylenol (TM) in a lifetime doubles the likelihood of kidney disease. Taking more than 5,000 NSAID pills *other than aspirin* also increases the incidence of kidney disease.[3] In addition, there are studies that have found a connection between NSAID usage and liver damage.[4]

The more powerful medications for arthritic diseases have even more powerful side effects. Corticosteroids, such as prednisone used in the treatment of rheumatoid arthritis, suppress the immune system. Long-term usage of corticosteroids has been correlated to increased incidence of bone fractures and cataracts.[7] Further, some of the more experimental drugs used in the treatment of some rheumatic diseases are close in function to those used in transplant operations that almost completely suppress the immune system.

Many of the drugs used in the treatment of the arthritic diseases interfere with the absorption of vitamins and minerals in the body. So not only are these medications adversely affecting various systems of the body, but they are also robbing the body of its essential nutritional building blocks for health and recovery.

---

[6] *Ibid.*, p. 30

[7] Ronco, P., and Flahault, A., "A Drug-induced End Stage Renal Disease," *New England Journal of Medicine,* Vol. 331, #25, 1994, p. 1711-1712

Surgery, including laminectomy of the spine and total joint replacement (as of the hip), are sometimes also resorted to when all other therapy has failed.

So what does Chinese medicine have to offer sufferers of arthritis?

Chinese medicine has two main things to offer sufferers of arthritis. The first is a whole range of natural treatments which help relieve pain but also promote healing of the tissues of the joints. These treatments include professionally prescribed and administered acupuncture and moxibustion, Chinese medical massage, and Chinese herbal medicine taken internally and used externally on the affected area. In addition, there are a number of highly effective, time-tested Chinese home remedies and self-treatments for joint pain.

Secondly, Chinese medicine has a much more down to earth and immediately understandable vision of what causes joint pain and what you can do for it. Most of us, on hearing that the most probable initial event in OA is the mitosis of the chondrocyte with increased synthesis of proteoglycans and type II collagen, won't have the foggiest notion of what this means on an everyday level and what we ourselves can do about this. Traditional Chinese medicine, on the other hand, is based on a vision of the human body as a microcosmic miniature of the natural world. Therefore, the language of Chinese medicine is the language we use every day to describe events in the world around us. More importantly, using this language, we are empowered to take charge of our own lives and well-being so that whether we experience pain and discomfort becomes a function of how we live our life.

So now, let's turn to how Chinese medicine describes and treats joint pain.

An Introduction to the Basic Concepts of Chinese Medicine

The Chinese medical term for all rheumatic diseases, including all types of arthritis, is *bi zheng*. This translates as "impediment condition." In Chinese medicine, *bi* or impediment means a blockage or obstruction that results in pain. A number of questions come to mind from this statement. What is being blocked or obstructed? How does this blockage or obstruction come about? And, probably the most important question, especially for people suffering with arthritis, what can be done to reduce or eliminate this pain? The remainder of this book will help you see how Chinese medicine answers these questions.

To understand how traditional Chinese medicine answers the above questions and treats rheumatic *bi* pain, we first need to discuss, describe, and explain the fundamental concepts of this oldest professionally practiced, literate, holistic medical system. As a system, Chinese medicine is logical. Based on its theories, a practitioner can perform treatments that achieve the desired effect. Therefore, it is also pragmatic and scientific in its own way. However, Chinese medicine is a separate system from modern Western medicine, and, as such, cannot be explained by Western medical words or logic. In other words, to truly understand the how and why of Chinese medicine, we need to approach it on its own terms.

When first hearing the theories and concepts of Chinese medicine, the reader may find them odd and mystifying. This is only natural when we begin to look at something that not only *appears different* but *is completely different than what we have been raised to believe as true and real*. As I tell my patients, if reality is what the vast majority of people agree to be true, then the Chinese medical view of the body and what causes disease must be "true and real." Over one billion people in Asia view the body and disease according to the ideas of Chinese medicine. However, more importantly, the fact that Chinese medicine has been effectively treating rheumatic *bi* conditions for over 2,000 years is what gives these ideas truth and reality.

Yin & yang

Yin and yang are the cornerstones for understanding, diagnosing, and treating the body and mind in Chinese medicine. In a sense, all the other theories and concepts of Chinese medicine are nothing other than an elaboration of yin and yang. Most people have probably already heard of yin and yang but may have only a fuzzy idea of what these terms mean.

The concepts of yin and yang can be used to describe everything that exists in the universe, including all the parts and functions of the body. Originally, yin referred to the shady side of a hill and yang to the sunny side of the hill. Since sunshine and shade are two interdependent sides of a single reality, these two aspects of the hill are seen as part of a single whole. Other examples of yin and yang are that night exists only in relation to day and cold exists only in relation to heat. According to Chinese thought, every single thing that exists in the universe has these two aspects, a yin and a yang. Thus every thing has a front and a back, a top and a bottom, a left and a right, and a beginning and an end. However, a thing is yin or yang *only in relation to its paired complement*. Nothing is in itself yin or yang.

It is the concepts of yin and yang which make Chinese medicine a holistic medicine. This is because, based on this unitary and complementary vision of reality, no body part or body function is viewed as separate or isolated from the whole person. The table

8

below shows a partial list of yin and yang pairs as they apply to the body. However, it is important to remember that each item listed is either yin or yang only in relation to its complementary partner. Nothing is absolutely and all by itself either yin or yang.

Yin	Yang
form	function
organs	bowels
blood	qi
inside	outside
front of body	back of body
right side	left side
lower body	upper body
cool, cold	warm, hot
stillness	activity, movement

As we can see from the above list, it is possible to describe every aspect of the body in terms of yin and yang.

Qi & blood

Qi (pronounced chee) and blood are the two most important complementary pairs of yin and yang within the human body. It is said that, in the world, yin and yang are water and fire, but, in the human body, yin and yang are blood and qi. Qi is yang in relation to blood which is yin. Qi is often translated as energy and definitely energy is a manifestation of qi. Chinese language scholars would say, however, that qi is larger than any single type of energy described by modern Western science. Paul Unschuld, perhaps the greatest living sinologist, translates the word qi as influences. This conveys the sense that qi is what is responsible for change and movement. Thus, within Chinese medicine, qi is that which motivates all movement and transformation or change.

In Chinese medicine, qi is defined as having five specific functions:

1. Defense

It is qi which is responsible for protecting the exterior of the body from invasion by external pathogens. This qi, called defensive qi, flows through the exterior portion of the body. The defensive qi plays an extremely important role in the development and the prevention of rheumatic *bi* conditions. As we shall see, when this qi is weak, external pathogens can enter and lodge in the body, especially in the joints, creating the blockage and obstruction that then develop into rheumatic *bi* conditions.

2. Transformation

Qi transforms substances so that they can be utilized by the body. An example of this function is the transformation of the food we eat into nutrients to nourish the body, thus producing more qi and blood.

3. Warmth

Qi, being relatively yang, is inherently warm. One of the main functions of the qi is to warm the entire body, both inside and out. If this warming function of the qi is weak, cold may cause the flow of qi and blood to be congealed similarly to the way cold effects water to produce ice.

4. Restraint

It is qi which holds all the organs and substances in their proper place. Thus all the organs, blood, and fluids need qi to keep them from falling or leaking out of their specific pathways. If this function of qi is weak, then problems like uterine prolapse, easy bruising, or urinary incontinence may occur.

5. Transportation

Qi provides the motivating force for all transportation in the body. Every aspect of the body that moves is moved by the qi. Hence the qi moves the blood and body fluids throughout the body. It is also qi which moves food through the stomach and the blood through its vessels.

Blood

In Chinese medicine, blood refers to the red fluid that flows through our vessels as recognized in modern Western medicine, but it also has meanings and implications which are different from those of modern Western medicine. Most basically, blood is that substance which nourishes and moistens all the body tissues. Without blood, no body tissue can function properly. In addition, when blood is insufficient or scanty, tissue becomes dry and withers.

Qi and blood are closely interrelated. It is said that, "Qi is the commander of the blood, and blood is the mother of qi." This means that it is qi which moves the blood but that it is the blood which provides the nourishment and physical foundation for the creation and existence of the qi.

In Chinese medicine, blood provides the following functions for the body:

1. Nourishment

Blood nourishes the body. Along with qi, the blood goes to every part of the body. When the blood is insufficient, function decreases and tissue atrophies or shrinks.

2. Moistening

Blood moistens the body tissues. This includes the skin, eyes, and ligaments and tendons of the body. Thus blood insufficiency can cause drying out and consequent stiffening of various tissues throughout the body.

3. Blood provides the material foundation for the spirit or mind.

In Chinese medicine, the mind and body are not two separate things. The spirit is nothing other than a great accumulation of qi. The blood (yin) supplies the material support and nourishment for the spirit (yang) so that it accumulates, becomes bright, and stays rooted in the body. If the blood becomes insufficient, the mind can "float," causing problems like insomnia, agitation, and unrest.

Essence

Along with qi and blood, essence is one of the three most important constituents of the body. Essence is the most fundamental material the body utilizes for its growth, maturation, and reproduction. There are two forms of this essence. We inherit essence from our parents and we also produce our own essence from the food we eat, the liquids we drink, and the air we breathe.

The essence which comes from our parents is what determines our basic constitution, strength, and vitality. We each have a finite, limited amount of this inherited essence. It is important to protect and conserve this essence because all bodily functions depend upon it, and, when it is gone, we die. Thus, the depletion of essence has serious implications for our overall health and well-being. Fortunately, the essence derived from food and drink helps to bolster and support this inherited essence. This is possible if we eat healthy and do not utilize more of our qi and blood than we create each day. Then, when we sleep at night, the surplus qi and especially the blood are transformed into essence.

The viscera & bowels

In Chinese medicine, the internal organs have a wider area of function and influence than in Western medicine. Each organ has distinct responsibilities for maintaining the physical health and psychological well-being of the individual. When thinking about the internal organs according to Chinese medicine it is more accurate to view an organ as a network that spreads throughout the body, rather than as a distinct and separate physical organ as described by Western science. In Chinese medicine, the relationship between the various organs and other parts of the body is made possible by the channel and network vessel system which we will discuss below.

Because the internal organs are conceived differently and perform different functions from their same named organs in modern Western medicine, they are referred to as the viscera and bowels. This is because, in Chinese medicine, there are five main viscera which are relatively yin and six main bowels which are relatively yang. The five yin organs are the heart, lungs, liver, spleen, and kidneys. The six yang bowels are the stomach, small intestine, large intestine, gallbladder, urinary bladder, and a system that Chinese medicine refers to as the triple burner. All the functions of the entire body are subsumed or described under these eleven viscera and bowels. Thus Chinese medicine *as a system* does not "have" a pancreas, a pituitary gland, or the ovaries. Nonetheless, the functions of these Western organs are described within the Chinese medicine system of the five viscera and six bowels.

The five viscera are the most important in this system. These are the organs that Chinese medicine says are responsible for the creation and transformation of qi and blood and the storage of essence. For instance, the kidneys are responsible for the excretion of urine but are also responsible for hearing, the strength of the bones including the low back, sexual reproduction, maturation and growth. This points out that the Chinese organs may have the same name and even some overlapping functions but yet are quite different from the organs of modern Western medicine. Each of the five viscera also has a corresponding tissue, sense, spirit, and emotion related to it. These are outlined in the table below.

Organ Correspondences

Organ	Tissue	Sense	Spirit	Emotion
Kidneys	bones/ head hair	hearing	will	fear
Liver	sinews	sight	ethereal soul	anger
Spleen	flesh	taste	thought	obsession/ worry
Lungs	skin/ body hair	smell	corporeal soul	grief/ sadness
Heart	blood vessels	speech	spirit	joy/fright

In addition, each viscus or bowel possesses both a yin and a yang aspect. The yin aspect of a viscus or bowel refers to its substantial nature or tangible form. Further, an organ's yin is responsible for the nurturing, cooling, and moistening of that viscus or bowel. The yang aspect of the viscus or bowel represents its functional activities or what it does. An organ's yang aspect is also warming. These two aspects, yin and yang, form and function, cooling and heating, create good health when they are in balance. However, if either yin or yang becomes too strong or too weak, the result will be disease.

The health of all five viscera is necessary for the prevention and/or the development of rheumatic *bi* problems. However, the viscera most directly related to rheumatic *bi* conditions are the kidneys, spleen, and liver. The involvement of these three viscera in rheumatic *bi* very dramatically illustrates the holistic nature of Chinese medicine. When these three viscera function properly and work together harmoniously, the body does not develop chronic rheumatic *bi* problems. If these three viscera do not function properly, then the body is at risk to develop acute and, eventually, chronic rheumatic *bi* problems.

In the remainder of this chapter we will describe the basic function of the kidneys, spleen, and liver. In the next chapter, we will see how these three viscera specifically relate to the condition of rheumatic *bi*.

The kidneys

In Chinese medicine, the kidneys are considered to be the foundation of human life. Because the developing fetus looks like a large kidney and because the kidneys are the main organ for the storage of inherited essence, the kidneys are referred to as the prenatal root. Thus it is essential to good health and longevity to keep the kidney qi strong and kidney yin and yang in relative balance. Exercises and lifestyle suggestions to develop, protect, and keep the kidneys robust are discussed in chapter 10.

The most important Chinese medical facts about the kidneys in terms of joint pain are:

1. The kidneys are responsible for human reproduction, development, and maturation. These are the same functions we described when we discussed the essence. This is because the essence is stored in the kidneys. Health problems related to reproduction, development, and maturation are commonly problems of kidney essence. Excessive sexual activity, drug use, or simple prolonged overexhaustion can all damage and consume kidney essence.

2. The kidneys rule the bones and marrow. This function includes the joints. Thus all chronic rheumatic *bi* problems involve the kidneys. Even if the disease did not start out affecting the kidneys, over time, chronic *bi zheng* will inevitably involve the kidneys. In Chinese it is said, "Enduring diseases will reach the kidneys." Conditions such as osteoporosis, degenerative disc disease and weak legs and knees also typically point to problems with the kidneys.

3. The kidneys are the foundation of water metabolism. They work in coordination with the lungs and spleen to insure that water is spread properly throughout the body and that excess water is excreted as urination. Therefore, problems such as edema, excessive dryness, or excessive day or nighttime urination can indicate a weakness of kidney function.

4. Kidney yin and yang are the foundation for the yin and yang of all the other organs and bowels and body tissues of the entire body. This is another way of saying that the kidneys are the foundation of our life. If either kidney yin or yang is insufficient, eventually the yin or yang of the other viscera and bowels will also become insufficient. The clinical implications of this will become more clear when we present rheumatic *bi* case histories.

5. The low back is the mansion of the kidneys. This means that, of all the areas of the body, the low back is the most closely related to the health of the kidneys. If the kidneys are weak, then there may be low back pain. For more information about Chinese medicine and low back pain see my book, *Low Back Pain: Care and Prevention with Traditional Chinese Medicine* also published by Blue Poppy Press.

The spleen

The spleen is the second most important yin viscus in rheumatic *bi* problems. The spleen and its paired bowel, the stomach, are central in the digestive process. The spleen plays a crucial role in the body's ability to transform food and drink into qi and blood. The spleen, kidneys, and lungs all play a part in the metabolism and movement of water throughout the body. However, the spleen plays the most crucial part when excessive body fluids gather and collect, transforming into dampness, as when the joints swell in RA. Readers familiar with Western anatomy and physiology may be scratching their heads as they compare the Chinese medicine ideas of spleen function with what they know the spleen does from Western physiology. Again, they should be cautioned that Chinese medicine views the internal organs and their functions differently from Western medicine.

Chinese medical statement of fact about the spleen in terms of joint pain include:

1. The spleen governs the transportation and transformation of food and water. This means that the spleen takes the partially digested food and fluids from the stomach and begins the process of transforming it into qi, blood, and essence. A healthy spleen is vital for producing sufficient qi and blood.

2. The spleen contains the blood. It is the spleen qi which holds the blood within its vessels. Therefore, if there is spleen qi vacuity, the person may experience various types of bleeding disorders or bruise easily.

3. The spleen governs the muscles and the four limbs. The muscles are dependent upon the spleen for their nourishment. If this spleen function is weak, the muscles will be weak and the legs and arms will lack power.

The liver

The liver is the third viscus in Chinese medicine frequently implicated in rheumatic *bi* conditions. While the bones and joints are related to the kidneys, the liver has a strong influence on the joints due to its control over the orderly spreading of the qi and its correspondence with the "sinews."

The basic Chinese medical statements of fact concerning the liver include:

1. The liver controls coursing and discharge. Coursing and discharge refer to the orderly spreading of qi to every part of the body. To be healthy, the qi needs to reach every part of the body. If the liver is not able to maintain the free and smooth flow of qi throughout the body, multiple physical and emotional symptoms can develop. This vital function of the liver is most easily damaged by emotional causes and, in particular, by stress and frustration. When we are frustrated, our qi wants to flow but the circumstances won't allow it. Usually, we repress our feelings in such instances and this then causes depression and constraint of the flow of qi controlled by the liver. This type of stagnation and constraint of the flow of liver qi due to emotional frustration and stress is called liver depression qi stagnation in Chinese medicine.

Liver depression qi stagnation can cause a wide range of health problems including PMS, chronic digestive disturbance, and depression and it can play a role in rheumatic *bi* conditions. Therefore, it is essential to keep the liver qi flowing freely. A number of effective ways to maintain a free flow of liver qi include deep relaxation and special exercises called *qi gong*. In chapter 10, I describe these and other ways to keep the liver qi flowing freely.

2. The liver stores the blood. This means that, when the body is at rest, the blood in the extremities returns to the liver. It is said in Chinese medicine that the liver is yin in form but yang in function. Thus the liver requires sufficient blood to keep it and its associated tissues moist and supple, cool and relaxed.

3. The liver controls the sinews. The sinews refer mainly to the tendons and ligaments in the body. Proper function of the tendons

and ligaments depends upon the nourishment of liver blood to keep them moist and supple. Chronic rheumatic *bi* problems often involve the tendons and ligaments surrounding the joints. Thus the connection between the tendons and ligaments and the liver's function of spreading the qi have implications for the treatment of chronic rheumatic *bi* pain. As we will see below, in all *chronic* rheumatic *bi* conditions, both the liver and the kidneys are believed to be insufficient and need to be supplemented.

The importance of the liver in terms of rheumatic *bi* complaints is explained by two of the above facts. First, the liver controls the smooth flow of qi throughout the body. If the liver is unable to maintain this free flow of qi there will be problems of stagnation and possibly blockage. Secondly, the liver has a close relationship with the blood. If the blood is insufficient, the sinews will become dry and unable to relax. In Chinese medicine blood has a close relationship with essence. It is said, "The blood and essence share a common source," and "the liver and kidneys share a common source." This means that blood insufficiency may lead to essence insufficiency and vice versa. It also means that liver disease eventually damages the kidneys. Thus many chronic conditions including chronic rheumatic *bi* problems involve both the liver and kidneys.

The channels & network vessels

Each viscus and bowel has a corresponding channel with which it is connected. In Chinese medicine, the inside of the body is made up of the viscera and bowels. The outside of the body is composed of the sinews and bones, muscles and flesh, and skin and hair. It is the channels and network vessels which connect the inside and the outside of the body. It is through these channels and network vessels that the viscera and bowels connect with their corresponding body tissues.

The channels and network vessel system is a unique feature of Chinese medicine. These channels and vessels are different from the circulatory, nervous, or lymph systems. The earliest reference to these channels and vessels is in *Nei Jing (Inner Classic)*, a text written around the 2nd or 3rd century BCE.

The channels and vessels perform two basic functions. They are the pathways by which the qi and blood circulate through the body and between the organs and tissues. Additionally, the channels connect the internal organs with the exterior part of the body. This channel and vessel system functions in the body much like the world information communication network. The channels allow the various parts of our body to cooperate and interact to maintain our lives.

The channel and network vessel system is complex. There are 12 so-called regular channels, six yin and six yang, each with a specific pathway through the external body and connecting with an internal organ (see diagram). There are also extraordinary vessels, channel sinews, channel divergences, main network vessels, and ultimately countless finer and finer network vessels permeating the entire body. All of these form a closed loop or circuit that is similar to, but energetically distinct from, the circulatory system of Western medicine.

Summary

By now you should have appreciation for and a basic understanding of the holistic nature of Chinese medicine. In Chinese medicine, nothing stands alone. Every part and function in the body *co-responds* to other parts and functions in the body. The body, mind, and spirit form an integrated whole. Health is the harmonious interaction of all the various aspects that comprise the organism. Disease and pain result when there is a disruption to this fundamental harmony and balance. In Chinese medicine, the focus of treatment is the restoration of harmony. Next, let's look at the cause of pain as we explore rheumatic *bi* conditions according to Chinese medicine.

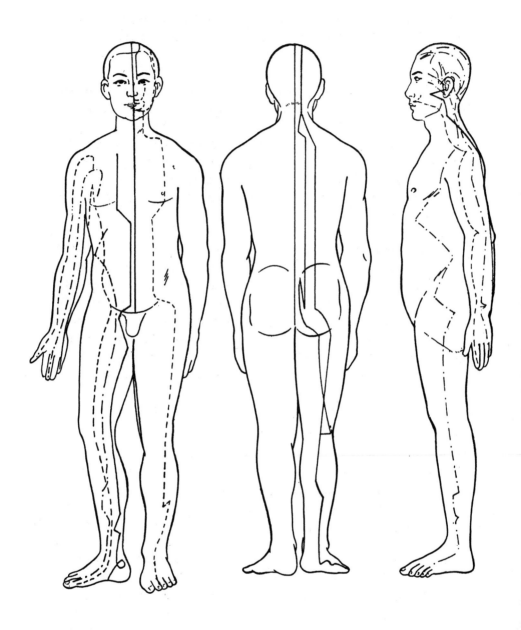

Pain According to Chinese Medicine

We have seen above that rheumatic complaints in Chinese medicine are classified as *bi*, and, whenever there is *bi* or impediment, there is pain. The following simple yet profound statement sums up the very essence of the Chinese medical view of pain:

If there is free flow, there is no pain;
If there is no free flow, there is pain.

This means that, as long as qi and blood flow freely and smoothly without hindrance or obstruction, there is no pain in the body. However, if, *due to any reason*, the flow of qi and blood is hindered, blocked, obstructed, or does not flow freely, then there will be pain. Thus, in Chinese medicine, pain is nothing other than the felt experience of lack of free flow of the qi and blood. As an extension of this, all joint pain is also nothing other than the experience of the lack of free flow of the qi and blood.

There are two main causes of the lack of free flow of the qi and blood. Either 1) something is hindering, blocking, or obstructing the smooth and uninhibited flow of qi and blood through the channels and vessels, or 2) there is insufficient qi and blood to maintain smooth and free flow. In the first case, lack of free flow is likened to a plug of hair and soap in a drainpipe. The water from the sink cannot flow freely because something is physically obstructing the pipe. In the second case, either there is insufficient qi to push the blood or insufficient blood to maintain uninterrupted flow. Just as a stream dries up in late summer and is eventually reduced to pools of disconnected water, these pools just sit and no longer flow together. This is like the lack of free flow due to insufficient blood.

All pain, no matter what its modern Western medical diagnosis, is considered by Chinese medicine as a problem with the free flow of qi and blood. Hence the Chinese medicine practitioner's job is to first diagnose the reason for the non-free flow of qi and blood and, second, to provide treatment which restores that free flow.

The flow of qi and blood can become inhibited in any and every area of the body: the internal organs, the muscles, the head, the low back, and the extremities and joints. For example, when we overeat and have acute indigestion with the accompanying sensations of abdominal fullness, bloating, and distention, these symptoms are due to the stagnation of stomach qi. In this case, the stomach qi cannot move freely through the excessive amount of food and drink in the stomach. Likewise, when we bruise ourselves and blood escapes from the blood vessels and then pools, we experience a mild form of blood stagnation, technically called blood stasis in Chinese medicine. In both these cases, the stagnation is not serious. We feel better within a short time and are free of symptoms when the qi and blood resume their proper functioning and flow freely.

According to Chinese medicine, the sensations of pain due to qi stagnation or blood stasis are different. Qi stagnation causes a feeling of distention or soreness that fluctuates in intensity and location. Qi stagnation pain often occurs with strong emotional changes. Blood stasis, on the other hand, is characterized by painful swelling or stabbing sharp pain at a specific, fixed location.

It is also possible for the qi and blood flow to become inhibited because of insufficiency of the qi, blood, or both. In this case, the pain is not severe but is enduring. If due to qi and blood insufficiency, the pain is worse after rest and better after light use. This is because, during rest or immobilization, there is insufficient qi and blood to keep the qi and blood moving. Movement itself helps to pump the qi and blood through the mobilized area. Therefore, movement tends to make this type of pain better.

If due primarily to qi insufficiency, then the pain is worse at the end of the day or after excessive exercise. In this case activity or exercise has used up the qi and left it even more deficient. Blood insufficiency pain tends to be worse at night after the scarce supply of blood has been consumed by the activities of the day and when it returns to the liver for storage.

In order for a Chinese medical practitioner to diagnose and treat rheumatic *bi* conditions, he or she must answer the following questions:

1. Is the pain due to blockage of the qi and blood or is it due more to the insufficiency of qi and blood?
2. If the pain is due to blockage, is the pain more characteristic of qi stagnation or blood stasis?
3. What pathogenic factors are causing the qi and blood stagnation?
4. What channels or network vessels are primarily involved in the pain?
5. What internal organs are involved?

The answers to these questions directly determine the treatment the patient will receive from their Chinese medical practitioner. The basic principle of treatment in Chinese medicine is to restore balance. Therefore, the *Nei Jing (Inner Classic)* says that, if a disease is due to too much of something, that something should be drained. If it is due to too little of something, that something should be supplemented. If it is due to heat, that heat should be cooled. If it is due to cold, that cold should be warmed. If it is due to dryness, that dryness should be moistened. And if it is due to dampness, that dampness should be dried.

In Chinese medicine, two patients with the same Western medical disease may receive radically different Chinese medicine treatments because the root cause of their disease is different. This means that every patient in Chinese medicine is given an individualized treatment based on the cause and nature of their particular pattern of disharmony.

The Four Basic Types of *Bi* Conditions

In the previous chapter, we saw that all pain is a reflection of a lack of free flow of either or both the qi and blood. We also saw that qi and blood may not flow freely because they either are blocked for some reason or there simply is not enough qi and blood to promote and maintain their flow. In Chinese medicine, rheumatic *bi* which is not associated with a known traumatic injury is typically ascribed to blockage by either wind, cold, dampness, or heat. These are the four basic types of *bi* conditions in Chinese medicine. In such cases, any one or a combination of two or more of these pathological energies may be lodged in the channels and network vessels where they are not supposed to be. In that case, the qi and blood which should be freely and smoothly flowing through those channels and vessels will not be able to. It is as if there were a traffic jam. Such pathological wind, cold, dampness, or heat may either invade the body from outside or, and especially in the case of dampness and heat, may be produced internally due to any of a number of factors.

External environmental pathogens

In Chinese medicine, there are three broad categories of disease causes. These are external causes, internal causes, and neither internal nor external causes. The external causes of disease are called external environmental excesses. There are six of these external environmental excesses or pathogens. They are wind, cold, dampness, heat, dryness, and summerheat. Any of these six factors may invade the body if either of two conditions exist. First, if one or more of these factors is unusually strong or unseasonable. For instance, very cold weather in the midst of summer or very warm weather in the midst of winter may allow these "excesses" to breach the body's defensive qi and invade. Secondly, if a person's defensive qi is weaker than it should be, any of these external pathogens if present in the environment may "take advantage of this vacuity, and enter." The *Nei Jing (Inner Classic)* says, "If evils enter, there must be vacuity." This implies that evils can enter only if the defensive qi is weaker than it should be. However, there are times when the external pathogenic qi in the external environment is so strong and virulent that it can breach the stoutest defense. This is then called epidemic or pestilential qi.

Internally engendered pathogens

Although wind, cold, dampness, and heat may all potentially invade the body from outside, three of these, cold, dampness, and heat may also be produced or engendered internally. If, for any reason, there is insufficient yang qi, the body will not be as warm as it should be. The absence of heat is none other than cold. Yang qi may be damaged by overexposure to a cold environment, in which case the body exhausts itself simply maintaining its body temperature. Yang qi may be damaged by overeating uncooked, chilled foods and drinking chilled liquids, since the process of digestion is the process of turning everything that goes into the stomach into 100°F soup. Yang qi may be damaged and depleted by any loss of yin fluids, since yin fluids are the foundation or root of yang qi. Such loss of yang fluids includes bleeding, massive sweating, unrelieved vomiting, unrelieved diarrhea, or continuous, unstoppable urination. And yang qi also becomes insufficient due to the decline of visceral function in turn due to aging. If the yang qi becomes insufficient to warm the body properly, it will not propel the blood and body fluids as it should. Instead, there is constriction and retardation of flow or *bi*.

Dampness may also be engendered internally due to any of several causes. Too much thinking and worry, overeating sweets, overeating damp-engendering foods, such as dairy products, wheat flour products, fruit juices, and oils and fats, and too little exercise may all damage the spleen. If the spleen is damaged and becomes weak and vacuous, then it will not move and transform body fluids properly. In that case, fluids will gather and collect and transform into dampness. Because dampness is a yin substance, it impedes the free flow of yang qi, thus resulting in *bi*. In addition, it is said in the *Nei Jing (Inner Classic)* that the spleen declines at around 35 years of age. Therefore, the spleen naturally weakens as a person ages. Consequently, one's ability to move and transform body fluids is not as good the older one gets past a certain age.

Likewise heat may be engendered internally. It does not have to invade from outside. In fact, in terms of rheumatic *bi* conditions, it relatively rarely does. In order to understand how pathological heat is engendered internally resulting in *bi*, one must understand that the body's healthy or correct qi (also called the righteous qi) is inherently warm in nature. If this qi backs up and accumulates for any reason, then this accumulated qi will manifest as heat. This is called transformative or depressive heat. It may be due to liver depression qi stagnation in turn transforming into depressive heat or it may be due to any other cause of blockage and obstruction. For instance, if dampness, blood, food, or phlegm gather and obstruct the free flow of yang qi, this may cause the accumulation of depressive or transformative heat. Therefore, in real life, given a sufficiency of righteous qi and either a long enough enduring or severe enough accumulation, damp *bi* and even cold *bi* may transform into heat *bi*.

Wind

Wind is usually the primary environmental factor to invade the body. Frankly, wind here does not mean physical wind. Rather, it only refers to an unseen pathogen which affects the body mysteriously and which provokes a series of responses in the body characteristic or reminiscent of the nature of wind. Thus, a person with a windy type of pain will feel discomfort that comes and goes and moves around the body from joint to joint. Just as wind moves about the earth, the person's complaints shift throughout the body. Because wind *bi*'s nature is changeable or movable, this type of impediment is also called movable *bi*. As mentioned above, in real life, wind as an external environmental pathogen typically combines with one of the other three. In Chinese medicine, the wind of wind *bi* is primarily seen as due to external invasion.

Cold

The emblem of cold in the natural world is ice, and, therefore, when cold causes *bi* or impediment, its nature and symptoms are reminiscent of ice. First, the pain of cold *bi* is worsened by exposure to cold and improved by warmth or heat. Secondly, because cold is so constricting to the flow of liquids, the pain tends to be quite intense. Therefore, cold *bi* is also called painful *bi*. And third, just as water becomes immobile when it turns to ice, so cold *bi* also tends to be fixed in location. Cold producing *bi* may be due either to external invasion or internal engenderment. When one says that someone is suffering from cold *bi*, all this really means is that the nature of their complaints share the characteristics of cold.

Dampness

Dampness is an accumulation of water or body fluids in the body. Because dampness is like a flood, the affected area is typically swollen and edematous. Because water tends to run downward, dampness tends to affect the lower part of the body more often than the upper part. Because water is heavy, damp *bi* tends to be stationary. It does not move around from joint to joint. It is worsened by exposure to dampness and may be improved when the weather or surroundings are clear and dry. In addition, dampness tends to be lingering. Typically, damp *bi* has a slow and insidious onset and then a long drawn-out course. And its pain is most often dull but persistent. Like cold above, dampness causing *bi* may be due to either invasion by external dampness or internally engendered dampness, with internal engenderment being the most common in the West.

Heat

Red is the color that corresponds to fire or heat in Chinese medicine. Therefore, when there is heat *bi*, the affected area is typically red. The area is usually also hot to the touch, and the pain is hot or burning in nature. As discussed above, heat *bi* or impediment is rarely due to external invasion of hot pathogens. Usually, heat *bi* is an acute exacerbation of other types of *bi*.

Qi Stagnation, Blood Stasis & Phlegm Nodulation

As we have seen above, most cases of rheumatic *bi* or impediment do involve wind, cold, dampness, and/or heat. This is why, in Chinese, the word rheumatic is translated as *feng shi*, wind dampness. However, whether these impediments are externally invading or internally engendered, they are often complicated by other factors involving the free flow of the qi and blood. Three of these factors are qi stagnation, blood stasis, and phlegm nodulation.

Qi stagnation

Qi stagnation is mostly due to emotional upset, stress, and frustration. Because of inability to fulfill one's desires, the liver qi cannot spread freely. This affects the liver's job of governing coursing and discharge. Because it is the qi which moves and transforms blood, body fluids, and food, if emotional upsetment and frustration cause liver depression qi stagnation, this then will affect the flow of qi and blood of the entire body and may lead to damp accumulation, phlegm obstruction, and/or food stagnation. In terms of joint pain, we already know that, "If there is pain, there is no free flow", and in the preceding chapter we have taken a look at the four main types of rheumatic *bi* conditions. Therefore, it is no wonder that liver depression qi stagnation often complicates and aggravates most, if not all, rheumatic *bi* complaints. On the one hand, the accumulation of dampness or heat in the body leading to impediment and, therefore, pain may be directly due to qi stagnation. On the other, if there is damp, blood, or phlegm depression in the body causing blockage and hindering free flow, this will eventually lead to or aggravate qi stagnation.

Blood stasis

Static blood, also called dead blood, malign blood, vanquished blood, and dry blood, means blood which is not moving. Rather, it obstructs the free flow of the channels and vessels the same way as silt obstructs the flow of a river or stream. Static blood may be due to traumatic injury. If traumatic injury severs the channels and vessels, the blood moves outside its vessels and then pools and accumulates. In other words, the blood can only keep flowing as long as it is inside its vessels. Once there is static blood, this yin accumulation then impedes the flow of qi and body fluids. This is why traumatic injuries are followed by swelling and inflammation. The vessels are severed and blood flows outside them. This static blood then impedes the flow of qi and body fluids. Body fluids gather and accumulate and there is edema. Qi, which is yang, accumulates and there is heat and redness or inflammation. Later, when the vessels are repaired, the qi moves the blood and body fluids through the vessels. Thus the swelling goes down, the redness and heat disappear, but the static blood which is left behind manifests as a "black and blue mark."

Because of the reciprocal relationship between the qi and blood, long-term qi stagnation will lead to blood stasis. As it is said in Chinese, "If the qi moves, the blood moves; if the qi stops, the blood stops." Therefore, anything which hinders and impedes the flow of qi will tend to eventually cause the complication of blood stasis. On the one hand, this means emotional upsetment and frustration. On the other, either externally invading or internally engendered *bi* will also, over time, tend to become complicated by blood stasis. Further, because the blood and body fluids flow together, if one of these gathers and collects, it will hinder and obstruct the free flow of the other. Thus dampness (or phlegm transformed out of dampness) over time will tend to become complicated by blood stasis, while long-term blood stasis will tend to become complicated by dampness and/or phlegm.

Phlegm nodulation

According to Chinese medical theory, phlegm is nothing other than accumulated dampness which has congealed into a thicker, denser form. Dampness may transform into phlegm if dampness simply endures for a long time. It may also congeal into phlegm due to either cold or heat. In the case of cold, it congeals dampness into phlegm like cold congeals water into ice. In the case of heat, it congeals dampness into phlegm like cooking pudding on a stove, the heat causing the fluids to thicken and condense. Once phlegm is produced, it obstructs and hinders the free flow of the qi, blood, and healthy body fluids. Such phlegm is typically produced by the internal organs, and especially the spleen which is in charge of moving and transforming body fluids. However, once produced, it often accumulates in the channels and vessels or in the space between the "muscles and flesh" and the "skin and hair." If it accumulates in either the channels and vessels or in the space between the muscles and skin, it may form into phlegm nodules, lumps of nonmoving, rubbery "phlegm." The nodulations associated with chronic, advanced rheumatic conditions are commonly considered, at least in part, phlegm nodulations in Chinese medicine.

Joint contracture & deformation

If *bi* or impediment persists in an area, it will prevent the local tissues from obtaining their proper nourishment. If the sinews fail to obtain their proper nourishment, especially blood, they will wither and dry out, thus contracting. Since the sinews in Chinese medicine refer to the tendons, ligaments, and other connective tissue, contracture of the sinews due to localized malnourishment leads to inability to flex and extend the affected joint(s). Likewise, enduring *bi* or impediment may prevent the bones from obtaining their proper nourishment. Thus the bones, *i.e.*, the heads of the bones, may become deformed. This process of deformation is accelerated or worsened if there is lingering heat impediment, in which case, pathological heat damages the bones.

Qi & Blood Vacuity

In Chinese medicine, it is believed that the spleen begins to decline some time in one's mid-30s due to aging. The spleen in Chinese medicine is the main viscus in charge of the production of qi and blood transformed for the food and drink we ingest. If there is insufficient qi and blood, it may result in joint pain due to two basic reasons. First, since the defensive qi which protects the exterior of the body from invasion by the six environmental excesses is also produced from the digestate, if there is spleen weakness and vacuity, there is also often a deficiency or insufficiency of defensive qi. In that case, the person is more easily invaded by the six environmental excesses, and we have seen that four of these may cause *bi* within the body: wind, cold, dampness, and heat. Secondly, if there is a spleen qi vacuity, there may not be sufficient qi to insure the movement of the blood and body fluids, while there may not be enough blood to nourish and maintain healthy, working sinews and vessels. Therefore, simply a lack of sufficient qi and blood may lead to a lack of free flow, not because of *bi* per se, but because there is not enough qi and blood to keep the qi and blood freely flowing.

Thus in Chinese medicine, there is the recognition that sometimes joint pain is not due to *bi*. Sometimes joint pain is due to simply a lack of sufficient qi and blood to keep the joints healthy and the qi and blood flowing freely. This is typically seen in older patients. Therefore, within Chinese medicine, there are the disease categories of "40 year shoulder" and "50 year wrist." In such cases, pain is typically worse after the person has been resting for some time. When we are at rest, our blood is stored in the liver and our qi is not mobilized to our extremities. Thus the sinews are less nourished and the qi and blood flow is not as free. When we try to use the joint after being at rest, at first it is sore and stiff. However, the movement itself promotes the flow of qi and blood. As the qi and blood flow more and more to and through the joint, the soreness and stiffness disappear.

However, in cases where there is little or no actual *bi* or impediment but soreness and stiffness is mainly due to insufficiency of qi and blood, too much exercise or overtaxation may also worsen the situation. All activity is nothing other than a consumption of qi and blood. Since activity itself consumes qi and blood the way a car consumes gasoline in order to operate, overconsumption, *i.e.*, overtaxation, will also lead to a worsening of any symptoms associated with insufficiency of the qi and blood. Therefore, while light exercise or mobilization relieves soreness and stiffness due to qi and blood insufficiency, heavy exercise or overtaxation make the situation even worse. Likewise, because qi and blood are consumed by living each day, such conditions are often worse in the evening or at night after we have consumed qi and blood all day long.

Spleen vacuity

We have seen that the spleen is the root of qi and blood production. We have also seen that the spleen declines and becomes weak due to age. However, spleen vacuity may also be due to overtaxation, excessive blood loss, too much thinking and worrying, and faulty diet. Since it is the spleen which plays the pivotal role in the production of qi, overconsumption of qi can wear out the spleen. Since it is the spleen that is the pivotal organ in the production of blood, excessive loss of blood can also wear out the spleen. For instance, since women lose blood on a monthly basis with their menstruation, they are more prone to spleen vacuity than men. This helps explain why women, or at least younger women, tend to have more systemic rheumatic complaints than men of the same age.

While too much thinking and especially worry and anxiety can damage the spleen, faulty diet is a main cause of spleen vacuity, particularly in the West. Overeating uncooked, chilled foods damage the spleen as does overeating sugars and sweets and damp, phlegm-producing foods. According to Chinese medicine, such damp-engendering, phlegm-producing foods include:

Milk	Wheat flour products
Cheese	Most fruits & fruit juices
Yogurt	Tomatoes
Oils & fats	Most nuts

If a person's spleen is vacuous and weak to begin with, these "heavy", harder to digest foods will overwhelm the spleen and damage it. In addition, they will tend to create or aggravate the presence of pathological dampness and phlegm. It is said in Chinese, "The spleen is averse to dampness." Therefore, faulty diet can cause or aggravate any case in which joint pain is associated with either qi and blood vacuity or the presence of dampness and phlegm. This includes a number of rheumatic diseases, including RA and systemic lupus erythematosus (SLE).

Kidney vacuity

The low back or lumbus is the "mansion" of the kidneys and the bones and joints are governed by the kidneys. This means that kidney vacuity weakness is often associated with low back soreness and pain as well as spinal column pain and deformation. In addition, because the kidneys begin to become weak after 40 years of age in most people due to the aging process, this also contributes to an increase of bone and joint problems after that age. In general, most people who have systemic diseases, such as RA and SLE, which have rheumatic pain as part of that disease do, according to Chinese medicine, have some element of spleen and/or kidney vacuity.

Treatment Based on Pattern Discrimination

In Chinese medicine, treatment is determined and given on the basis of the patient's pattern and not simply on the basis of their named disease. A Chinese medical pattern is different from the patient's named disease. And, in professionally practiced Chinese medicine, treatment is given primarily based on the pattern and only secondarily on the patient's disease diagnosis. Thus it is said in Chinese:

> One disease, different treatments.
> Different diseases, same treatment.

This means that two patients may receive very different Chinese medical treatments *if their Chinese patterns are different*, while two patients with different named diseases may receive the same treatment *if their Chinese patterns are the same*. For example, a patient with rheumatic *bi* due to wind, cold, and dampness with spleen yang vacuity will receive a completely different treatment from a patient with rheumatic *bi* with kidney yin vacuity. While both patients could have the identical Western medical diagnosis of rheumatoid arthritis, each would have two totally different sign and symptom complexes from the Chinese medical point of view. Therefore, each would be treated according to their own particular pattern. Because Chinese medicine treatments are based upon identifying an individual's unique pattern, Chinese medicine causes no side effects or other medically induced problems.

A person's Chinese pattern takes into account all the signs and symptoms of the disease plus all the patient's other, seemingly unrelated, signs and symptoms *and* the Chinese description of the cause of their condition. Therefore, all the person's symptoms are noteworthy, not just the ones that are specific to the major complaint. In fact, the Chinese medicine practitioner gathers so much information, the patient may not see the relevance of it all. A typical first interview may take from 45 minutes to 2 hours in order to gather all the necessary information for a comprehensive assessment. Certainly the Chinese medicine practitioner takes much more time to ask questions about all aspects of the person's life in contrast to the 15 minute exam common with the typical Western MD.

As we have seen in the previous chapters, rheumatic *bi* conditions are due to a lack of free flow of the qi and/or blood due to impediment by wind, cold, damp or heat as well as qi stagnation, blood stasis, phlegm nodulation, qi and blood vacuity, and vacuities of the spleen and kidneys. Hence, there are a number of different factors accounting for any given person's individualized rheumatic complaints. This means that, in Chinese medicine, each patient with a rheumatic complaint or some sort of joint pain will receive their own, uniquely tailored treatment plan in turn based on their unique pattern of disharmony. It is only by obtaining *all* the person's signs and symptoms that the practitioner can begin to identify all the factors that contribute to this individual's rheumatic *bi* condition.

How Chinese medicine patterns are determined

How does a Chinese medical practitioner determine the pattern of disharmony that is causing an individual's rheumatic *bi* condition? First, the practitioner must have a good understanding of the theories of Chinese medicine. This includes an in-depth knowledge of qi and blood, viscera and bowels, channels and network vessels, and yin and yang and how these interconnect and interact. Secondly, the practitioner must understand how illness develops and how injury affects the body. Third, the patterns of illness that develop due to external invasion, internal damage, or traumatic injury must be understood and discriminated. Keeping all of this theoretical information in mind, the practitioner then obtains information from the patient.

The four examinations

Since before the time of Christ, Chinese medical practitioners have used what are called the four examinations for obtaining information about a patient's condition. These four examinations are 1) looking, 2) listening/smelling, 3) asking, and 4) touching.

1. Looking focuses on what the practitioner can see with their unaided eyes (except for normal corrective lenses). Everything about the patient that can be observed can be useful. This includes their facial expression, the brightness of their eyes, their facial complexion, bodily constitution, posture and manner of movement, inspection of the affected area, and examination of the tongue and its coating.

Tongue diagnosis is a highly developed skill in Chinese medicine and a major source of information about a patient's condition. Both the tongue itself and its coating are indicators of the person's condition. For example, a thick, greasy, yellow tongue coating indicates the presence of damp heat, while a shiny, red tongue without a coating indicates a yin vacuity.

2. Listening and smelling are the second method of examination in Chinese medicine. The character in the Chinese language for this examination means both listening *and* smelling as a single concept. (This underscores that Chinese medicine divides up the pie of reality in a very different way than how we do in English.) The practitioner listens to the patient's breathing, the quality of their voice, or other sounds, such as a cough. For example, a person with a weak voice who coughs when active may have weak

qi. Body odors and the smells of any excretions also give the practitioner useful information about the patient's pattern.

3. Questioning the patient is the third method of examination. These questions include when and how the problem happened, how long it has gone on, what treatment has already been given and with what results, general medical history, sensations of cold and heat, location and quality of pain, descriptions of urination and bowel movements, sleep patterns, perspiration, headaches, dizziness, appetite, thirst, digestive disturbances, energy level, gynecological problems, and more. Because the sensations of pain due to stagnation of qi and blood differ as do the pain and aching due to the various types of *bi*, the patient's description of the pain is critical in determining what type of *bi* or what type of pattern exists.

4. The last examination method is touching. Some Chinese medical practitioners consider this the most important of the four methods when it comes to rheumatic *bi* conditions. Only by touching various areas of the body can the practitioner directly know the condition of the body and its internal organs.

The most important aspect of this method, at least in terms of assessing viscera and bowel function and basic quantities and qualities of qi and blood flow, is taking the pulse. Together with the information gained from examining the tongue, taking the pulse is central to Chinese medical diagnosis. Chinese pulse diagnosis requires great skill and sensitivity. The pulse taken at the wrist provides information about the basic state of the person's qi and blood, yin and yang, viscera and bowels, and pathogenic factors. There are 28 different standard pulse qualities described in the classical literature. For example, people in pain who have a lot of qi and blood typically have a pulse which is tight "like a taut rope", while people in pain with less qi and blood typically have a pulse which is wiry "like the string of a zither."

By gathering information through the four examinations and by comparing the patient's signs and symptoms with the condition of the tongue and pulse, the patient's pattern is understood and named. The name of the pattern describes an inherent state of imbalance. For instance, kidney yin insufficiency means that kidney yin is too weak. Therefore, the next step is creating a treatment plan which will correct the imbalance implied in the name of the pattern. If there is kidney yin vacuity, the kidneys should be supplemented and yin should be nourished or enriched. Hence treatment techniques are applied to bring about this result, the return to balance and, therefore, health.

Chinese Treatment Methods for Rheumatic *Bi*

Once a professional practitioner of Chinese medicine has determined the person's individualized pattern of disharmony, they then formulate a treatment plan. In other words, having figured out what is wrong, the practitioner is faced with the question, "What corrective measures need to be applied to promote healing in this person?" In terms of the professional Chinese medical treatment rheumatic *bi* conditions, there are four main treatment modalities or methods. These are acupuncture, moxibustion, Chinese herbal medicine, and Chinese medical massage.

Acupuncture & moxibustion

When the average Westerner thinks of Chinese medicine, they probably first think of acupuncture. Certainly acupuncture is the best known of the various methods of treatment which go to make up Chinese medicine. However, in China, acupuncture is actually a secondary treatment modality, most Chinese immediately thinking of "herbal" medicine when thinking of Chinese medicine.

Be that as it may, most professional practitioners of Chinese medicine in North America are licensed or otherwise registered and permitted to practice medicine as acupuncturists. Therefore, most such practitioners treat every patient with at least some acupuncture no matter if they also prescribe a Chinese herbal formula as well.

What is acupuncture?

Acupuncture primarily means the insertion of extremely thin, sterilized, stainless steel needles into specific points on the body where Chinese doctors have known for centuries there are special concentrations of qi and blood. Therefore, these points are like switches or circuit breakers for regulating and balancing the flow of qi and blood over the channel and network system we described above. As we have seen above, the pain experienced as an integral part of rheumatic *bi* complaints is due to a loss of free flow of the qi and blood. Since acupuncture seeks to directly and immediately regulate the flow of qi and blood through the channels and vessels, acupuncture is an especially good treatment option for eliminating *bi* pain. In China, acupuncture is so well known for its effective treatment of all sorts of *bi* conditions that the treatment of rheumatic complaints makes up the major part of most acupuncturists' practices.

As a generic term, acupuncture also includes several other methods of stimulating acupuncture points, thus regulating the flow of qi in the body. The main other modality is moxibustion. This means the warming of acupuncture points mainly by burning dried, aged Oriental mugwort on, near, or over acupuncture points. The purpose of this warming treatment are to 1) even more strongly stimulate the flow of qi and blood, 2) add warmth to areas of the body which are too cold, and 3) add yang qi to the body to supplement a yang qi vacuity. Because the warmth of moxibustion is an immediate and specific remedy for cold *bi*, moxibustion is almost always used to treat that kind of impediment. However, because moxibustion does move the qi and quicken the blood more powerfully than acupuncture, it is also used to treat non-cold *bi* which is enduring or recalcitrant, *i.e.*, stubborn, to treatment. Since Chinese doctors typically do not add heat to heat, moxibustion is not ordinarily used for treating heat *bi*.

Other acupuncture modalities are to apply suction cups over points, to prick the points to allow a drop or two of blood to exit, to apply magnets to the points, to warm the points with various types of heat lamps, and to stimulate the points by either electricity or laser.

What is a typical acupuncture treatment like?

In China, acupuncture treatments are given every day or every other day, three to five times per week depending on the nature and severity of the condition. In general, it is best if one can get acupuncture every day for the first couple of treatments if arthritis or other joint pain is really severe. Once the pain has diminished some, one can begin to space out the treatments to every other day and thence to once or twice a week. After four to five weeks, the treatments should be tapered off completely. As a general rule, the longer a condition has lasted, the longer treatment also usually lasts. A basic rule of thumb is to allow one month of treatment for every year a condition has persisted. However, it is also possible for even a long-standing condition to completely disappear after only one or two treatments.

When the person comes for their appointment, the practitioner will ask them what their main symptoms are, will typically look at their tongue and its fur, and will feel the pulses at the radial arteries on both wrists. Then, they will ask the patient to lie down on a treatment table. Based on their Chinese pattern discrimination, the practitioner will select anywhere from one to eight or nine points to be needled. Some of these needles will be inserted near to or surrounding the affected joint, while others of these needles will probably be inserted at points located at some distance from the actual place of pain. These "distant" points, nevertheless, are connected to the site of pain by the Chinese channels and network vessels.

The needles used today are ethylene oxide gas sterilized disposable needles. This means that they are used one time and then thrown away, just like a hypodermic syringe in a doctor's office. However, unlike relatively fat hypodermic needles, acupuncture needles are hardly thicker than a strand of hair. The skin over the point is disinfected with alcohol and the needle is quickly and deftly inserted somewhere typically between one quarter and a half inch. In some few cases, a needle may be inserted deeper than that, but most needles are only inserted relatively shallowly.

After the needle has broken the skin, the acupuncturist will usually manipulate the needle in various ways until he or she feels that the qi has "arrived." This refers to a subtle but very real feeling of resistance around the needle. When the qi arrives, the patient will usually feel a mild, dull soreness around the needle, a slight electrical feeling, a heavy feeling, or a numb or tingly feeling. All these mean that the needle has tapped the qi and that treatment will be effective. Once the qi has been tapped, then the practitioner may further adjust the qi flow by manipulating the needle in certain ways, may attach the needle to an electroacupuncture machine in order to stimulate the point with very mild and gentle electricity, or they may simply leave the needle in place. Usually the needles are left in place from 10-20 minutes. After this, the needles are withdrawn and thrown away. *Thus there is absolutely no chance for infection from another patient.*

Does acupuncture hurt?

In Chinese, it is said that acupuncture is *bu tong*, painless. However, most patients will feel some mild soreness, heaviness, electrical tingling, itching, or distention. When done well and sensitively, it should not be sharp, biting, burning, or really painful.

Ear acupuncture

Acupuncturists believe there is a map of the entire body in the ear and that by stimulating the corresponding points in the ear, one can remedy those areas and functions of the body. Therefore, many acupuncturists will not only needle points on the body at large but also select one or more points on the ear. Ear acupuncture is especially good for relieving many types of body pain. Hence, ear acupuncture can be a real boon for sufferers of rheumatic *bi* pain.

The nice thing about ear acupuncture points is that one can use tiny "press needles" which are shaped like miniature thumbtacks. These are pressed into the points, covered with adhesive tape, and left in place for five to seven days. This method can provide continuous treatment between regularly scheduled office visits. Thus ear acupuncture is a nice way of extending the duration of an acupuncture treatment. In addition, these ear points can also be stimulated with small metal pellets, radish seeds, or tiny magnets, thus getting the benefits of stimulating these points without having to insert actual needles.

Chinese herbal medicine

The repertoire of healing ingredients used in Chinese medicine includes more than 5,000 substances. Since the majority of these are from vegetable sources, these medicinals are often referred to as "herbs" even though, in some cases, this is a misnomer. Each of these medicinals has a specific action on the body. For example, there are medicinals that dispel wind, and scatter cold. Others move the qi and quicken the blood. While yet others may supplement the kidneys and nourish the liver or enrich yin and clear heat. Typically, these medicinals are combined into multi-ingredient formulas meant to rebalance the pattern of imbalance the patient presents. These formulas may contain anywhere from four to twenty-four or more ingredients, and a number of Chinese herbal formulas have been successfully used for centuries to treat rheumatic *bi* conditions.

Such formulas are most commonly administered in the form of water-based, oral decoctions. A decoction is the technical name for a liquid extract made by boiling medicinals in water, removing the dregs, and administering the remaining medicinal liquid. However, Chinese medicinals are also administered in the form of pills, powders, alcohol-based tincture and "wines", and as teas and porridges internally. Externally, they may be used in the form of poultices, plasters, compresses, liniments, washes, and soaks.

While rheumatic *bi* conditions can often be very adequately treated by acupuncture and moxibustion alone, if the condition involves vacuity weakness of any of the viscera, such as the spleen or kidneys, or if there is persistent heat which must be cleared, acupuncture is usually more effective when combined with Chinese herbal medicine. This is because the needles cannot really add any qi or blood to the body, while there are Chinese medicinals which can supplement or add to the body's qi and blood. Likewise, although acupuncture can often reduce inflammation locally, when one of the viscera or bowels is chronically overheated, Chinese herbal medicine taken internally is often a quicker and more efficient method of treatment. In addition, phlegm nodulation usually requires internal medicinal treatment and blood stasis certainly benefits from Chinese herbal medicine.

Chinese medical massage

Chinese medical massage is called *tui na* in Chinese. This means to push and grasp. However, Chinese medical massage is made up of a number of other massage manipulations besides pushing and grabbing. In fact, medical massage has been developed into a high art in China, and there is typically a separate ward or clinic devoted to its practice in every medium and large Chinese medical hospital in China. Although each different "stroke" or manipulation is meant to achieve a very specific therapeutic effect, in general, Chinese massage is, like acupuncture and moxibustion, meant to directly and immediately free and regulate the flow of qi and blood in the channels and vessels. Because its effect on the qi and blood flow is so immediate, Chinese medical massage is an important method in the treatment of any condition, such as *bi*, where there is a lack of free flow.

The above four methods may be applied either individually or together. Many Western practitioners of Chinese medicine are trained to practice all four modalities. Therefore, depending on the patient's pattern of illness and other factors, a patient might receive a combination of all four modalities. However, some practitioners only practice acupuncture and moxibustion, while others practice only *tui na*. What combination of therapies the practitioner decides to use in treatment of each individual patient depends on the individual practitioner's training, clinical experience, and personal preference. In addition, there are a number of minor treatment modalities that are also often employed as an adjunct to acupuncture and moxibustion. These include cupping, small hammers with and without tiny needles embedded in their heads for percussing the skin, magnets, and heat lamps. Further, some acupuncturists stimulate the acupuncture points electrically, with lasers, or with colored light. Again, all these variations depend on the practitioner's training and inclination and the patient's pattern and condition.

Case Histories

One of the best ways to get a good picture of how Chinese medicine works is through the presentation of case histories. Case histories take the reader from initial examination through treatment to final outcome. Since Chinese medicine is a dynamic system meant to be put to pragmatic use in the real world, seeing it in action is the best and most accurate way to understand it. Therefore, a number of case histories are described below. Each case history exemplifies the diagnosis and treatment of one of the major Chinese medical patterns associated with joint pain and rheumatic complaints.

These case histories show how each person's rheumatic pain fits into a Chinese medicine pattern which is holistic when compared with a Western medical rheumatic disease diagnosis. The signs and symptoms in these cases take into account everything about each patient. Thus you will see how a pattern is determined and a treatment plan is developed that aims at healing *all the patient's signs and symptoms*, not just the major rheumatic complaint. In other words, these case histories show how Chinese medicine treats the whole person at the same time as their rheumatic pain.

Early stage rheumatic pain

Wind damp exterior pattern

Kurt, age 27, was camping in the mountains over the weekend and was caught in a spring rainstorm while hiking. The next day, he awoke with a headache, a bit of a chill, slight fever, and his body "felt really heavy and sore all over, especially in the joints." When I inspected his tongue, it was a normal color with normal, thin, white fur. When I felt his pulse, it was floating and bowstring. Kurt contracted a wind damp condition in the superficial aspect and muscles of his body. The headache, heaviness of his body, and sore joints are indicative of pain due to damp *bi*. When dampness blocks the free flow of qi, there is achy pain. Conditions with sudden onset typically indicate that wind is involved. "Wind" is the vector that commonly carries the other five environmental excesses into the body. In this case, damp was, therefore, combined with wind. The chills, slight fever, normal tongue and fur, and the floating pulse all indicated that he had an "exterior" condition. The bowstring pulse indicates that his qi is not flowing freely.

Kurt's treatment included both acupuncture and Chinese herbal medicine to release or resolve the exterior portion of his body and to dispel the invading pathogenic factors of wind, eliminate dampness and stop pain. Acupuncture consisted of needling *Fu Liu* (Ki 7) and *He Gu* (LI 4), *Feng Men* (Bl 12) and *Feng Chi* (GB 20), and *Kun Lun* (Bl 60). The first two points promote perspiration, thus relieving the exterior and kicking the wind back out of the body. The second two points are called "wind" points. In particular, they treat pain in the upper back, head, and neck due to external invasion of wind. While the last point is a point which releases the entire back of the body. It is used when an external pathogen has lodged in the most superficial layer of the body resulting in pain.

In terms of Chinese herbal medicine, I prescribed *Qiang Huo Sheng Shi Tang* (Notopterygium Overcome Dampness Decoction), a standard formula for wind damp *bi* due to exterior invasion. It consisted of Radix Et Rhizoma Notopterygii (*Qiang Huo*), Radix Angelicae Pubescentis (*Du Huo*), Radix Et Rhizoma Ligustici (*Gao Ben*), Radix Ledebouriellae Divaricatae (*Fang Feng*), Radix Ligustici Wallichii (*Chuan Xiong*), Fructus Viticis (*Man Jing Zi*), and mix-fried Radix Glycyrrhizae (*Gan Cao*). These medicinals were boiled in three cups of water down to 1 ½ C of liquid. The dregs were removed and Kurt was instructed to drink ½ C three times that day. The next day, Kurt called me to say that he was feeling much better. The fever and chills had disappeared, his body no longer felt heavy, and his joint pain was gone. On follow-up two weeks later, Kurt said that there had been no further complications.

Wind damp heat exterior pattern

Alice, age 26, had felt bad for two days. She had back pain, fever, slight chills, an achy feeling in her body, and red, swollen knees that felt hot to the touch. Her tongue was slightly red at the tip and had slightly yellow fur. Her pulse was floating, bowstring, and rapid. Alice had contracted a wind damp heat condition. Alice's recent onset of fever and chills indicated the presence of an external factor that was still in the superficial part of her body. The fever and red-hot knees indicated the presence of heat. The swollen knees indicated the presence of dampness. The body achiness and leg pain was due to blockage of qi by this external dampness impediment. The red-tipped tongue and yellow fur indicated pathogenic heat, while the floating pulse confirmed an exterior pattern, the bowstring pulse confirmed that the qi was not flowing freely, and the rapid pulse confirmed the presence of pathological heat.

Like Kurt, Alice received an acupuncture treatment and some Chinese herbs. However, her acupuncture consisted of *He Gu* (LI 4) and *Wai Guan* (TB 5), *Du Bi* (St 35) and *Nei Xi Yan* (M-LE-16a), and *Yang Ling Quan* (GB 34) and *Yin Ling Quan* (Sp 9). The first two points in this formula clear heat and resolve the exterior. The second pair treat knee pain by freeing the flow locally. And the last pair also treat the local flow of qi at the same time as clearing heat and eliminating dampness from the body in general.

The herbal formula Alice received contained Cortex Phellodendri (*Huang Bai*), Semen Coicis Lachryma-jobi (*Yi Yi Ren*), Rhizoma

Atractylodis (*Cang Zhu*), Radix Achyranthis Bidentatae (*Niu Xi*), Radix Stephaniae Tetrandrae (*Han Fang Ji*), Radix Gentianae Macrocephalae (*Qin Jiao*), and Fructus Chaenomelis Lagenariae (*Mu Gua*), medicinals which clear heat, dispel wind, eliminate dampness, and eliminate impediment specifically from the lower limbs.

The next day, Alice reported that the acupuncture treatment had really helped reduce the knee pain almost immediately. The feverish feeling was gone, but the knees still felt a little hot to the touch and there was still a little bit of "hot" pain in the knees. Therefore, I refilled the same prescription and instructed Alice to take it another two days to make sure she recuperated completely. By the end of that time, the pain and hot feelings were eliminated. On follow-up after two weeks, there had been no recurrence.

Both Alice's and Kurt's rheumatic pains were clearly acute conditions. Both were of sudden onset which is one indication of invasion by wind. The fever and chills they each experienced are also a primary indicator of a superficial invasion of the body by external pathogens. According to Chinese medicine, invasions by environmental excesses first attack the exterior part of the body, that is the skin and muscles.

Kurt and Alice both were wise to seek such immediate professional treatment. Chinese medicine strongly advises that superficial illness be quickly and properly resolved. If the environmental factors are not dispersed and eliminated through either proper treatment or the body's own healing forces, they can lodge in the channels and become the cause of chronic rheumatic/arthritic conditions. Remember, the longer a pathogenic factor blocks the flow of the qi and blood through the body, the more difficult it is to eliminate. Therefore rheumatic *bi* conditions, like all life's challenges and problems, are best resolved early before they become more troublesome.

However, we are not always successful in taking care of and eliminating problems when they first arise. We often let things go, including illnesses. We hope they will sort themselves out and, with time, just go away. Sometimes this approach to life works. Often, illnesses and health problems do resolve themselves without intervention. In those cases, the natural healing ability of the body is at work. However, sometimes, this approach does not work. Some illnesses progress and, rather than go away, become chronic.

Let's now look at what happens when a rheumatic condition progresses beyond initial invasion as seen in our above two cases. First, this means that there are no longer the symptoms of superficial invasion, *i.e.*, fever and chills. However, in some cases, the person may have fever accompanying their rheumatic pain. This type of fever is now due to heat that is being internally generated. Secondly, the cases that follow could now be classified as true rheumatic conditions or *bi* conditions in Chinese medicine. Here, the environmental factors, wind, cold, and damp or wind, heat, and damp, are now lodged in the channels traversing the joints or other areas of the body, blocking the flow of qi and blood and thus causing pain.

Chronic rheumatic pain

Wind, cold, damp *bi*

Tom was in his early 50s and worked as an area consultant for a multilevel marketing company. When he arrived for his first appointment, he had difficulty walking due to the pain in his left knee. He also had pain in the right elbow and left shoulder. The pain was aggravated by changes in the weather, especially rain and cold. His joints felt cold to the touch and were stiff. The only times he felt "normal" was when he soaked in a hot tub. These hot soaks would ease his pain for an hour or two.

Tom had been playing softball in a gentle rain four months previous. He had gotten "chilled to the bone." That evening, he developed some sniffles and continued to feel chilled. For the next several days, he had felt achy all over and then the pain "just settled into my joints." He had hoped it would go away, but it hadn't.

Tom's condition was due to wind, cold, and damp. Whereas, in Kurt and Alice's cases described above, the invasion of external environmental excesses were resolved without further complication, Tom had developed an early stage rheumatic *bi* condition.

The original sniffles, chill, and achiness were symptoms of wind, cold, damp invasion. The continued joint pain indicated that the pathogenic factors wind, cold, and dampness had now lodged in the channels. The joint stiffness that got worse with rain, indicated the presence of damp. Changes in the barometric pressures that accompany the arrival of a new weather front can also make damp conditions worsen. The pain relief he experienced by soaking in a hot tub as well as the sensation of cold in his joints indicated the presence of cold. From a Western medical perspective, Tom's condition could indicate early stage rheumatoid arthritis, osteoarthritis, or bursitis.

Tom was treated by a combination of acupuncture, moxibustion, and Chinese medicinals. The focus of treatment was to dispel the wind, scatter the cold, eliminate the dampness, and circulate the qi and blood through the channels traversing his painful joints. Points were needled around each joint as well as distant points on the channels along which the pain was felt. While the needles were in place, moxa (Folium Artemisiae Argyii, *Ai Ye*) was attached to and burned on the heads of the needles surrounding the affected joints. This is called warm needle technique. Tom received three treatments the first week, two treatments each the second and third weeks, and one treatment during week four. During this entire course of treatment, he also took the Chinese herbal patent medicine, *Guan Jie Yan Wan* (Close Down Joint Inflammation Pills), eight pills each time, three times per day. These pills treat joint pain due to wind, damp, cold *bi*. Between office visits, Tom was given some Chinese medicinal plasters to apply externally to the most painful joints. These were called *Shang Shi Zhi Tong Gao* (Damage by Dampness, Stop Pain Plasters). Using the above-mentioned modalities, Tom's pain was completely eliminated within one month.

Tom's condition was an early stage rheumatic wind, damp, cold *bi*. He had no symptoms or signs of weakness in any of his internal organs. Therefore, the treatment focused upon removing the pathogens lodged in the channels traversing his painful joints. It is important to keep in mind that patients with a long-standing rheumatic *bi* condition will often show symptoms of spleen vacuity and/or dampness, liver depression and/or vacuity, and kidney yin and/or yang vacuity weakness. In such cases, the imbalance within the internal organ(s) must be addressed if the condition is to completely resolve and the cure be long lasting. The focus of treatment in these cases must include treating the affected organ(s) as well as removing the impeding factors that are blocking and hindering the free flow of qi and blood. Below are a number of cases that demonstrate the importance of treating the internal organs at the same time as addressing the rheumatic joint pain.

Chronic wind, cold, damp *bi* with a predominance of wind

Phyllis, 57, loved to run and hike. However, for the past three years, she'd dramatically reduced her activities due to pain in her elbows, knees, and neck. Her Western MD had diagnosed osteoarthritis and suggested she take NSAIDs (non-steroidal anti-inflammatory drugs) to control the pain. During Phyllis's Chinese medical exam, she said her pain had a tendency to move from joint to joint and varied from a sharp to a dull, achy sensation. "Some days my knees hurt; other days it's my neck or my elbows." She reported occasional numbness in the muscles of her forearms.

Her pains tended to worsen under strong wind conditions which occurred frequently at her home in the foothills of the Rocky Mountains. Phyllis's low back was also achy and sore. She liked warmth and felt "a bit better" when the weather was warm. Phyllis loved the mountains so much that moving to a warmer, less windy climate was not a consideration.

Phyllis"s Chinese medical diagnosis was wind, cold, damp *bi* with a predominance of wind, along with kidney vacuity. Two of Phyllis"s symptoms were indicative of pain due to wind. When pain moves from joint to joint as it did in Phyllis's case, it is like the wind moving from place to place. Pains that change in quality, sometimes dull sometimes sharp, are also indicative of pathogenic wind. The presence of cold was indicated by the fact that Phyllis deliberately sought warmth and found it effective in reducing her pain. Her low back pain was a sign that her kidneys were weak. This was corroborated by the fact that she got up two times to urinate each night, that her feet were particularly cold, and that her libido was almost nonexistent. In addition, her age suggested kidney vacuity as well, since the kidneys typically become vacuous and weak by or after the late 40s in women. The numbness in her forearm was due to the blockage of the qi and blood. It is said in the *Nei Jing (Inner Classic)* that the tissues can function and feel when they obtain blood to nourish them. When the tissues are not properly nourished, numbness, *i.e.*, lack of sensitivity, may occur.

Phyllis also received acupuncture, moxibustion, and Chinese herbal medicine to dispel wind, scatter cold, and eliminate dampness. However, her treatment also included strengthening her kidneys and, in particular, kidney yang. In this case, the predominate pathogenic factor was wind, but this was combined with kidney vacuity weakness. Acupuncture and moxibustion (warm needle technique) was used to eliminate the pathogenic factors, while Chinese medicinals were used to strengthen the kidneys and the liver. In this case, Phyllis was prescribed the Chinese patent medicine, *Du Zhong Feng Shi Wan* (Eucommia Wind Damp Pills), four pills each time, two times per day. These pills not only include ingredients to dispel wind, scatter cold, and eliminate dampness but also to supplement the kidneys and invigorate yang.

The kidneys are the foundation of the yin and yang. It is also said that, "enduring disease (eventually) reaches the kidneys." When the kidneys are weak, the liver is also often weakened, especially in postmenopausal women. In Phyllis's case, there were no signs of liver weakness. However, a Chinese medical practitioner always keeps in mind that the liver "shares a common source" as the kidneys. In addition, the liver is responsible for nourishing the sinews, *i.e.*, ligaments and tendons, which are important tissues in all joints. The liver is also involved in insuring that the qi flows smoothly through the body. Thus, for all joint problems, it is important that the kidneys and the liver are healthy and functioning properly.

In Phyllis's case, we see two important principles in the treatment of rheumatic *bi* conditions according to Chinese medicine. First, we must determine what pathogenic factors are involved and in what proportion. In Phyllis's case, pathogenic wind was the most prominent pathogen. Knowing this, the practitioner can tailor the treatment to primarily dispel wind. There are specific acupuncture points and specific medicinals that dispel wind, just as there are specific acupuncture points and medicinals to scatter cold, eliminate dampness, or clear heat. Secondly, it is essential to determine the strength of the internal organs. If the internal organs are weak, as is often the case in chronic conditions, it will be difficult, if not impossible, for treatment to succeed. In Phyllis's case, the kidneys needed to be strengthened to insure her recovery.

Wind, cold, damp *bi* with a preponderance of cold

Ralph, 59, needed to take an early retirement from his job as a plumber after he had been diagnosed with osteoarthritis. He had intense, sharp pains in his neck, shoulders, and hands with a decrease in range of motion. He hated the cold because it made his pain worse. His painful joints were cold to the touch and so was his abdomen. Ralph also tended to have loose stools.

Ralph, like Phyllis above, had a wind, damp, cold *bi* condition. But the major pathogen in Ralph's case was cold. Pain due to cold is intense, sharp, or even stabbing. This is due to the fact that cold blocks the flow of qi and blood the same way that cold freezes water into ice. When cold is the predominant pathogenic factor in an impediment condition, the person does not tolerate cold weather well. Cold weather "adds" to the existing cold in the channels, thus causing even more stagnation of qi and blood and thus increasing the already intense pain. Ralph's tendency toward loose stools and abdominal coldness indicated that his spleen, specifically his spleen yang, was also weak. Loose stools, especially after meals and/or containing undigested food, are a major symptom of spleen vacuity. When a person has loose stools, a feeling of coldness, and the abdomen is cold to the touch, it is a sure indicator that the warming aspect of the spleen, that is the yang, is weak.

Cold rheumatic *bi* conditions are treated by using warmth to scatter cold and warm yang. Ralph's treatment consisted of acupuncture, moxibustion, and Chinese herbal medicinals to warm the channels, scatter cold, and warmly supplement spleen yang. Moxibustion is an essential component in the treatment of pathogenic cold in the channels and helps to warm and fortify spleen yang. Ralph was given a moxibustion stick for home use so he could give himself daily treatments to warm the channels and the spleen. In addition, he was prescribed *Xiao Huo Luo Dan* (Small Quicken the Network Vessels Elixir), a Chinese medicine which primarily treats cold *bi*. This was accompanied by another Chinese patent medicine, *Xiang Sha Liu Jun Zi Tang* (Auklandia & Amomum Six Gentlemen Pills), the most famous Chinese formula for spleen vacuity loose stools.

Two days after beginning treatment, Ralph began to feel better. His joints began to feel warmer and the pain was considerably reduced. Ralph was directed to eat cooked foods and refrain from eating uncooked vegetables and fruits and chilled, iced, or frozen foods and drinks as these foods and beverages only add cold to cold and thus easily damage spleen yang. In Ralph's case, we wanted to protect and warm his spleen yang to disperse the cold that had accumulated in his neck, shoulders, and arms.

Two cases of painful swollen red knees

The next two cases demonstrate how important it is in Chinese medicine to see rheumatic conditions holistically. At first glance, both individuals appear to have the same problem. Both have a red, painful, swollen knee. However, as we shall see, the causes are very different, and, therefore, the treatments for these two patients is also very different. If the same Chinese medical treatment were administered to both individuals, one of them would recover, while one would get much worse.

Craig was in his early 40s and worked as a computer pro- grammar. He loved his work because he did not need to interact with many people. As he so politely put it, "I'm a very irritable person. An SOB." For the past two years, his right knee was very painful. "It will blow up like a balloon and get really red and hot. Most of the time, it's just a little swollen and red." He'd tried a number of medications for his knee that helped for a short while but did not completely get rid of the pain. He came to see me to see if a more holistic approach to his problem might help.

Craig loved to put ice on his knee and, in fact, felt best when he soaked in a cold tub, even in winter. He hated summer because the heat was just too much. He drank ice water "by the gallon" daily even in the winter and had a red face. He tended toward being constipated.

Craig is a classic case of damp heat *bi*. The swollen knee is a sign of pathogenic dampness. Signs of heat included irritability (*i.e.*, heat affecting the Chinese medical idea of the liver), redness in the knee and face (red is the color of heat in Chinese medicine), thirst for cold beverages (heat damages and consumes body fluids and, therefore, causes a desire for cold drinks), and constipation (if the intestines are dried out by pathogenic heat, the stools will be too dry to move). In Craig's case, the heat was due to internal causes. There were no signs or symptoms such as fever and chill to indicate that he had had an external invasion. In addition, there was no history of the condition being initiated by an external pattern. His preference for cold, the use of ice on the knee, the cold soaks, and love of winter are all further evidence that Craig is systemically too hot.

Craig was treated by a combination of acupuncture and Chinese herbal medicine. He was prescribed the same formula as Alice above. However, to this formula, Radix Et Rhizoma Rhei (*Da Huang*) and Mirabilitum (*Mang Xiao*) were added to purge the bowels and clear heat specifically from the large intestine (and therefore also from the liver according to Chinese medical theory). This formula relieved Craig's constipation at the same time as it reduced the pain and inflammation in his knee. Because there already was too much heat, moxibustion was not used at all. Craig needed to be treated for two months before his knee pain went away entirely. To this day, if Craig overeats hot, peppery, greasy, oily, spicy foods and drinks too much alcohol, twinges of pain and his constipation return. In that case, he knows immediately to change to what Chinese medicine calls a "clear, bland diet" and to purge his bowels with Milk of Magnesia. He has not had to receive any further acupuncture in several years.

Jan was also in her early 40s. She was a grade school teacher who loved her work. However, for the past year, her right knee was bothering her more and more. She'd had pain in her knee for many years following a skiing injury. Initially, her knee was swollen without redness. For the past few months, the knee was both swollen, red, and hot, especially after a long week on her feet. Jan was easily chilled and loved warmth. "It can never be too warm for me." The thought of putting ice on her knee was not appealing even though it was hot to the touch. She tended to have swelling in her feet (edema) along with loose stools and occasional low back pain.

Jan's knee pain was due to long-standing wind, cold, and damp *bi* transforming into a wind, damp, heat *bi* condition. Over time and given the right bodily constitution and conditions, some patient's wind, cold, damp rheumatic *bi* will transform into a heat *bi* condition. This is what had happened to Jan. Her original cold, damp knee problem was now a localized damp heat problem. Unlike Craig above, Jan's swollen, red-hot knees were the only heat signs and symptoms she had. Everything else pointed to a cold and damp condition. Her love of warmth and dislike of cold and her loose stools indicated vacuity cold due to a weakness of her spleen yang. The swelling of the knee and the edema in the feet were signs of excessive dampness in her body. In fact, Jan's cold, damp constitutional condition was due to a weakness of her kidney and spleen yang, the edema being due to both the spleen and kidneys being too weak to move and transform body fluids properly, while the low back pain was a classic kidney vacuity symptom in a woman her age.

Therefore, when it came to treatment, Jan received the same herbal formula as Alice and Craig. However, unlike Craig, Radix Et Rhizoma Rhei and Mirabilitum were not added. Instead, this formula was combined with the Chinese patent medicine *Shen Ling Bai Zhu Pian* (Ginseng, Poria & Atractylodes Tablets), a well-known formula for treating spleen vacuity. Although only acupuncture was used locally in order to drain off the depressed qi (*i.e.,* heat) and move the dampness, moxibustion was applied to the points on the back which supplement the spleen and kidneys (*Pi Shu*, Bl 20, and *Shen Shu*, Bl 23, respectively). In addition, moxibustion was also performed at *Guan Yuan* (CV 4) and *Zhong Wan* (CV 12), one on the lower abdomen and the other on the upper abdomen, in order to also help supplement and warm the kidneys and spleen. Eight acupuncture treatments were sufficient to eliminate the red, swollen, painful knees. At that point, the herbal formula in decoction was discontinued as was the insertion of needles around the knees. However, Jan's husband was taught how to do the moxibustion on her back and abdomen in order to continue supplementing the kidneys and spleen for two months more. Likewise, she took the Chinese pills until her stools were no longer loose.

In both these cases, Craig and Jan complained of the "identical" problem of painful, red, swollen knees. Yet when we look beyond the knees to what is taking place in the rest of the body, we see that these individuals have very different internal conditions. What they share in common is that both needed to have damp and heat cleared and eliminated from the channels that traverse the knee in order to cure the knee redness, swelling, and pain. However, in Craig's case, internal heat also needed to be cleared, while in Jan's case, internal vacuity cold needed to be supplemented and warmed. If the treatment that was administered to Craig was given to Jan, she would have gotten worse. Her weakened kidney and spleen yang would not have been able to handle the heat-clearing medicinals that Craig needed and was able to handle. Likewise, the treatment Craig received would have further weakened Jan's kidney and spleen yang causing her to feel even colder, exacerbating her loose stools (possibly causing diarrhea) and creating even worse swelling in the legs which would have increased her knee pain.

Two cases of rheumatoid arthritis

The next two cases of rheumatoid arthritis also demonstrate how the same presenting problem, when looked at from the Chinese medical perspective, can have two very distinct and different causes which require two different approaches to treatment.

Cold in the channels with blood weakness

Rosa was a thin, athletic 29 year-old, single accountant who had received a positive diagnosis of rheumatoid arthritis (RA) the previous year. While Western medications were able to control her pain, she was worried about the long-term adverse effects on her health of using medications. A friend suggested she try Chinese medicine to see if it could help.

Rosa reported that her fingers would occasionally feel a little stiff. She had no bony changes in her hands or fingers. Since beginning the Western medications, the pain had been eliminated. Rosa's major complaint, beyond her diagnosis of RA and her stiff fingers, was her cold hands and feet. These were cold to the touch and had been so since her teenage years. Upon inquiry, it was found that she suffered from long menstrual cycles with sparse blood flow, dry skin, nails that easily split, and hair that was dry and "felt lifeless."

According to Chinese medicine, Rosa's diagnosis was accumulation of cold in the channels with blood vacuity. Rosa had no yang vacuity symptoms like those of Jan above who had cold along with kidney and spleen yang vacuity. Rosa's symptom of long menstrual cycles with little blood indicated she had blood vacuity, especially in light of her other blood vacuity symptoms. The blood is responsible for nourishing the skin, hair, and nails. When the blood is vacuous and insufficient, the skin can be dry, the nails can easily split and crack, and the hair can lack luster and life. Because the blood was so vacuous and insufficient, it was also not able to nourish her extremities. Thus cold was able to accumulate in the channels at the same time as her sinews became dried out due to malnourishment. The cold had caused her pain, but this had been eliminated by the Western medication. The remaining stiffness was a sign of stiff, dry sinews in turn due to blood vacuity.

In this case, Rosa was given a famous Chinese herbal formula for nourishing and supplementing the blood. Called *Si Wu Tang* (Four Materials Decoction), its main ingredients are Radix Angelicae Sinensis (*Dang Gui*), cooked Radix Rehmanniae (*Shu Di*), Radix Albus Paeoniae Lactiflorae (*Bai Shao*), and Radix Ligustici Wallichii (*Chuan Xiong*). All these ingredients supplement and nourish the blood in Chinese medicine. To these, Caulis Milletiae Seu Spatholobi (*Ji Xue Teng*) was added to even more effectively nourish the blood while at the same time quickening the blood and eliminating any residual cold dampness. In addition, Radix Astragali Membranacei (*Huang Qi*) was added to boost the qi. It takes qi to engender and transform the blood. Therefore, adding a qi-supplementing ingredient can make the blood-nourishing medicinals work more quickly.

Rosa noticed a change in her stiff fingers within three days of beginning this formula. Her menses came earlier than she expected and the flow was heavier and longer. After taking this formula for two months, she reported her nails no longer cracked and that her hair also seemed fuller and healthier. Since acupuncture cannot directly nourish the blood, no acupuncture was necessary, but this case would have been hard to treat without the Chinese herbal medicine.

Damp *bi*

Ken, 42, had been diagnosed with RA two weeks previous to our first meeting. An obese man, he was very anxious about his ability to continue his work as a graphic artist. The fingers on both hands were slightly swollen, stiff, and sore. This made working as an artist difficult. Images of his aunt's crippled fingers haunted him. He experienced increased discomfort on cloudy, cold, rainy days. He had a numb and heavy sensation in both arms. When asked to describe his diet, he turned beet red. "I live on junk food." Breakfast and lunch consisted of food purchased at a fast food restaurant. Supper, which he ate with his wife, was a "traditional American meal": a main course of meat with some vegetable and bread followed by a sugary desert. Ken's tongue was swollen and contained the imprints of his teeth on its borders, while its fur was thick, white, and slimy looking. Ken's pulse was soggy and bowstring.

Ken"s diagnosis was wind, cold, damp rheumatic *bi*. The primary pathogen was dampness. When damp settles into the channels, there will be stiffness, possible swelling, a heavy sensation, and possible numbness. A further indicator of Ken's problem with damp was his weight, since, in Chinese medicine, fat is considered a problem of excessive dampness and phlegm. In addition, Ken's swollen, edematous tongue showed that he was not moving and transforming body fluids properly. The thick, white, slimy tongue fur showed that there was an accumulation of dampness, stagnant food, and possibly phlegm clogging his system. The soggy pulse showed that Ken's spleen was weak and that dampness was spilling over into the spaces between his muscles and flesh and his skin. This was obstructing the flow of qi and blood and so gave the pulse an image of constraint, a bowstring pulse.

Because, Ken's dampness was due to poor spleen function in turn due to faulty diet, I instructed Ken on the principles of a clear, bland diet high in complex carbohydrates and fresh vegetables and low in sugars and sweets, dairy products, oils and fats, and uncooked and/or chilled foods and beverages. I also instructed Ken on the importance of regular exercise. I treated Ken's sore, stiff, swollen fingers with acupuncture twice a week for several weeks. In addition, I prescribed a Chinese herbal formula which primarily supplemented the spleen and eliminated dampness.

Ken is still overweight and still does not eat what Chinese medicine would call a perfect diet. When work gets really stressful, Ken typically "does not have time to eat right." When that happens, his fingers swell up and become stiff and sore. When Ken eats right and gets regular exercise, he has no symptoms of his RA. During acute episodes, Ken runs back in to see me again. I do a couple of acupuncture treatments on his hands and give him another pep talk about diet and exercise. Otherwise, Ken is able to take care of himself and has continued to be able to practice his profession very successfully.

According to Western medicine, both Ken and Rosa had the same disease, rheumatoid arthritis. From the Chinese medical point of view, they had two completely different problems which required different treatments. Both patients were encouraged to incorporate a number of self-care suggestions into their daily routines. Rosa and Ken were encouraged to regulate their diets using the guidelines outlined in chapter 10. They were advised to eat a more vegetarian diet and to eat primarily cooked foods. Both patients needed to improve their diets to strengthen their spleens. The spleen is responsible for the formation of blood (which was vacuous and insufficient in Rosa) and for moving and transforming dampness (which was excessive in Ken).

Conclusion

The cases presented above are but a sample of the complex spectrum of rheumatic diseases and the role Chinese medicine can play in their treatment. It is hoped that by reading these case histories and the multiple symptoms that accompany each person's pain that you now have a feel for how a practitioner of Chinese medicine weaves together the many and various signs and symptoms to form a complete picture of the person—their Chinese medical pattern as opposed to their disease.

When talking with a prospective patient on the phone, I often suggest that the person write an "obsessive" list of all their health problems and complaints. Problems that seem unrelated to the patient's disease may be relevant to a practitioner of Chinese medicine in determining the patient's pattern. In the case of recent injuries, the Chinese medical practitioner will primarily focus on the injury itself and may not concern themselves overly much with all the other signs and symptoms. However, when dealing with stubborn, chronic conditions, every detail of the patient's bodily functions is important in making the overall pattern discrimination. Western patients used to seeing highly specialized Western M.Ds typically need to be reminded that their Chinese medical pattern is the sum total of all their signs and symptoms, even mental and emotional ones.

That is the beauty of Chinese medicine. It does not just treat individual symptoms or individual diseases. It treats the whole person, for the Chinese pattern is nothing other than a snapshot of the whole person, body and mind. Thus good quality, professional Chinese medicine relieves the major complaint and, in doing so, also improves the health of the entire person. Because each and every one of its treatments takes into account their effect on the total pattern, Chinese medicine heals without iatrogenesis (*i.e.*, doctor-caused disease) or side effects.

While Chinese medicine cannot reverse the damage done to the bony structures of the body as seen in advanced cases of osteo- and rheumatoid arthritis, it can reduce the person's pain and suffering and help prevent further deterioration. As mentioned above, the sooner a painful joint condition is treated, the easier it is to help restore the person to health and improved functioning. If you or someone you know are currently suffering from a rheumatic condition, I urge you to consider trying Chinese medicine to reduce your pain and improve your health.

The Three Free Therapies for Arthritis and Rheumatic Complaints: Diet, Exercise & Deep Relaxation

When first practicing Chinese medicine, a patient said, "I want you to fix me." Since then, I have had many patients who have repeated that same phrase word for word. My standard response to that request is, "You fix a machine. The body heals."

Most readers of this book have grown up under the care of Western medicine with the attitude that it is the physician's job to "fix" what is wrong. The doctor's responsibility is to diagnose and prescribe medication, and the patient's responsibility is to take the medicine. Little or nothing more is asked of the patient. When the symptoms go away, we believe the "problem is fixed" and we resume business as usual.

This "fix it" approach certainly appears to work for certain health problems, such as surgery for appendicitis. In such a situation, there is minimal patient involvement in the recovery process with little need to make lifestyle changes. However, this method of health care is a set up for the person who "comes down with" a disease or medical condition that does not lend itself to an easy fix. Even when there is no quick fix or magic bullet, patients often persist in pursuing a medicine that can simply get rid of their problem, refusing to believe that there isn't such a medicine. In Western industrial nations, we harbor the illusion that professional medical intervention by itself is all that is necessary to make our illness go away, and quickly.

75

It can be a shock for many Western patients to learn that many conditions of ill health require us to make changes in how we live in order to recover. People with heart conditions awaken to this reality when they learn they need to alter their diet, increase their exercise, and learn to manage their stress more effectively. In other words, they need to change *how* they live if they want to continue to live.

The same advice is applicable to those individuals who suffer from chronic rheumatic conditions. If you truly want to live with less pain, you need to change how you live. The following two chapters are written to help you bring about the necessary changes so that you can have less pain, become more functional, and reduce your reliance upon medications.

Creating the conditions of healing

I find the phrase, "creating the conditions of healing", helps people understand that they need to take an active role in their own health care. "Creating the conditions of healing" is like gardening. When we garden, we need to create a number of conditions so that our seeds will grow. First, we need to turn the soil over and fertilize it. Then we need to make sure that the garden gets the proper amount of sun for the types of plants we are cultivating. We need to plant the seeds at the right depth. We need to make certain that the seeds get enough water, but not too much. If these conditions are met, then we have done our job as gardener well. We've done everything possible to create the right conditions for the seeds to sprout and grow. At this point in the process, we wait for the miracle of life to unfold. All gardening, after the planting time, is waiting. We wait to see the plants poke through the soil. At that point, no amount of impatience, anger, or demanding can change the outcome of our garden. And finally, when the sprouts appear, we need to protect them from the wild world of weeds, birds, insects, and all the other things that will do them harm.

Likewise, we are the gardeners of our own life. We need to plant the seeds of healthy habits that promote healing in our own life. We need to nurture these wholesome habits and protect ourselves from those behaviors that destroy our garden. If we create the proper conditions in our life, then it is possible for the healing power of the body to take over. Moment by moment, we are either creating the conditions of healing or we are creating the conditions that have gotten us to the point of pain and disease.

It can be helpful to visualize our life and the many elements that compose our life as a daisy. Each petal is an aspect of our life. To create the conditions of healing we must make certain that each of the petals is well cared for. In this chapter, we will explore the healing benefits of the three free therapies: diet, exercise, and deep relaxation. Then, in the next chapter, we will explore a number of self-help therapies.

Diet

In Chinese medicine, digestion is primarily the function of the spleen and stomach, and, therefore, Chinese dietary therapy mostly has to do with promoting the healthy function of these two organs. The function of the spleen and stomach are likened to a pot on a stove or still. The stomach receives the foods and liquids which then "rotten and ripen" like a mash in a fermentation vat. The spleen then cooks this mash and drives off (i.e., transforms and upbears) the pure part. This pure part collects in the lungs to become the qi and in the heart to become the blood. All the principles of Chinese dietary therapy, including what persons with rheumatic complaints should and should not eat, are derived from these basic "facts."

77

Because the spleen is the root of qi and blood engenderment and transformation, keeping the spleen functioning properly helps insure sufficient constructive and defensive qi. If the defensive qi is sufficient, it will secure the exterior of the body against invasion by the six environmental excesses. If the constructive and defensive qi are both sufficient, then the body will be properly warm. Since warmth is one of the factors which promote and allow for the free flow of the qi and blood, sufficient qi to warm the body is important in preventing inhibited flow of the qi and blood due to cold.

Secondly, healthy spleen function insures the blood production is sufficient. If the spleen does not engender and transform sufficient blood, then the tissues of the body, including the sinews, will not receive adequate nourishment. If the sinews do not receive adequate nourishment, they dry up and become stiff. This then leads to stiffness and limitation in the range of movement of the joints surrounded by the sinews.

Third, the spleen is in charge of moving and transforming body fluids. If the spleen becomes diseased and loses control over this function, fluids will collect and gather, transforming into dampness. Dampness may then spill over into the space between the muscles and skin, impeding the free flow of the qi and blood through the channels and vessels. Although dampness is one of the six environmental excesses, dampness causing rheumatic *bi* conditions in the West is rarely due to external dampness alone. Further, if dampness endures for a long time or is transformed by either cold or heat, it may congeal into phlegm. Since phlegm is even denser than dampness, phlegm hinders and obstructs the free flow of qi even more than does dampness, and in Chinese medicine it is said, "the spleen is the root of phlegm engenderment."

Fourth, because all the viscera and bowels of Chinese medicine form a single, interdependent whole, the function of the spleen is intimately connected to the function of all the other viscera and bowels. In particular, healthy spleen function insures healthy liver and kidney function. If the spleen is strong and sufficient, then this helps the liver maintain its control over coursing and discharging, which, in turn, helps insure the free flow of qi throughout the body. Mostly this ability of the spleen to control the liver has to do with the spleen's engendering sufficient blood to emolliate and harmonize the liver. Because spleen qi and kidney yang are interdependent, spleen vacuity will eventually "reach" the kidneys, leading to kidney yang vacuity. Since the kidneys govern the bones and joints, kidney vacuity can either cause or aggravate many types of joint pain. Although the spleen and kidneys both become debilitated by age (usually first the spleen and that leading to the kidneys), the spleen is the easier of the two viscera to supplement and strengthen via the diet. Conversely, damage of the spleen due to faulty diet can speed up and exacerbate weakness and vacuity of the kidneys.

Therefore, it is easy to see that a healthy, functioning spleen is of utmost importance to the prevention and treatment of all joint pain and rheumatic conditions. When it comes to Chinese dietary therapy and the spleen, there are two main issues: 1) to avoid foods which damage the spleen, and 2) to eat foods which help build qi and blood.

Foods which damage the spleen

In terms of foods which damage the spleen, Chinese medicine begins with uncooked, chilled foods. If the process of digestion is likened to cooking, then cooking is nothing other than pre-digestion outside the body. In Chinese medicine, it is a given that the overwhelming majority of all food should be cooked, *i.e.*, predigested. Although cooking may destroy some vital nutrients (in Chinese, qi), cooking does render the remaining nutrients much more easily assimilable. Therefore, even though some nutrients have been lost, the net absorption of nutrients is greater with cooked foods than raw. Further, eating raw foods makes the spleen work harder and thus wears the spleen out more quickly.

If one's spleen is very robust, eating uncooked, raw foods may not be so damaging, but we have already seen that many women's spleens are already weak because of their monthly menses overtaxing the spleen *vis a vis* blood production. It is also a fact of life that the spleen typically becomes weak with age.

More importantly, chilled foods directly damage the spleen. Chilled, frozen foods and drinks neutralize the spleen's yang qi. The process of digestion is the process of turning all foods and drinks to 100° Fahrenheit soup within the stomach so that it may undergo distillation. If the spleen expends too much yang qi just warming the food up, then it will become damaged and weak. Therefore, all foods and liquids should be eaten and drunk at room temperature at least and better at body temperature. The more signs and symptoms of spleen vacuity a person presents, such as fatigue, chronically loose stools, undigested food in the stools, cold hands and feet, dizziness on standing up, and aversion to cold, the more closely she should avoid uncooked, chilled foods and drinks.

In addition, sugars and sweets directly damage the spleen. This is because sweet is the flavor which inherently "gathers" in the spleen. It is also an inherently dampening flavor according to Chinese medicine. This means that the body engenders or secretes fluids which gather and collect, transforming into dampness, in response to foods with an excessively sweet flavor. In Chinese medicine, it is said that the spleen is averse to dampness. Dampness is yin and controls or checks yang qi. The spleen's function is based on the transformative and transporting functions of yang qi. Therefore, anything which is excessively dampening can damage the spleen. The sweeter a food is, the more dampening and, therefore, more damaging it is to the spleen.

Another group of foods which are dampening and, therefore, damaging to the spleen is what Chinese doctors call "sodden wheat foods." This means flour products such as bread and noodles. Wheat (as opposed to rice) is damp by nature. When wheat is steamed, yeasted, and/or refined, it becomes even more dampening. In addition, all oils and fats are damp by nature and, hence, may damage the spleen. The more oily or greasy a food is, the worse it is for the spleen. Because milk contains a lot of fat, dairy products are another spleen-damaging, dampness-engendering food. This includes milk, butter, and cheese.

If we put this all together, then ice cream is just about the worst thing a person with a weak, damp spleen could eat. Ice cream is chilled, it is intensely sweet, and it is filled with fat. Therefore, it is a triple whammy when it comes to damaging the spleen. Likewise, pasta smothered in tomato sauce and cheese is a recipe for disaster. Pasta made from wheat flour is dampening, tomatoes are dampening, and cheese is dampening. In addition, what many people don't know is that a glass of fruit juice contains as much sugar as a candy bar, and, therefore, is also very damaging to the spleen and damp-engendering.

Below is a list of specific Western foods which are either uncooked, chilled, too sweet, or too dampening and thus damaging to the spleen. Persons with rheumatic pain should minimize or avoid these proportional to how weak and damp their spleen is.

Ice cream
Sugar
Candy, especially chocolate
Milk
Butter
Cheese
Margarine
Yogurt
Raw salads
Fruit juices
Juicy, sweet fruits, such as oranges, peaches, strawberries, and tomatoes
Fatty meats
Fried foods
Refined flour products
Yeasted bread
Nuts
Alcohol (which is essentially sugar)

If the spleen is weak and wet, one should also not eat too much at any one time. A weak spleen can be overwhelmed by a large meal, especially if any of the food is hard-to-digest. This then results in food stagnation which only impedes the free flow of qi all the more and further damages the spleen.

A clear, bland diet

In Chinese medicine, the best diet for the spleen and, therefore, by extension for most humans, is what is called a "clear, bland diet." This is a diet high in complex carbohydrates such as unrefined grains, especially rice, and beans. It is a diet which is high in *lightly cooked* vegetables. It is a diet which is low in fatty meats, oily, greasy, fried foods, and very sweet foods. However, it is not a completely vegetarian diet. Most women, in my experience should eat one to two ounces of various types of meat two to four times per week. This animal flesh may be the highly popular but over-touted chicken and fish, but should also include some lean beef, pork, and lamb. Some fresh or cooked fruits may be eaten, but fruit juices should be avoided. In addition, women should make an effort to include tofu and tempeh, two soy foods now commonly available in North American grocery food stores.

If the spleen is weak, then one should eat several smaller meals than one or two large meals. In addition, because rice 1) is neutral in temperature, 2) fortifies the spleen and supplements the qi, and 3) eliminates dampness, it should be the main or staple grain in the diet.

A few problem foods

Coffee

There are a few "problem" foods which deserve special mention. The first of these is coffee. Many people crave coffee for two reasons. First, coffee moves stuck qi. Therefore, if a person suffers from liver depression qi stagnation, temporarily coffee will make them feel like their qi is flowing. Secondly, coffee transforms essence into qi and makes that qi temporarily available to the body. Therefore, people who suffer from spleen and/or kidney vacuity fatigue will get a temporary lift from coffee. They will feel like they have energy. However, once this energy is used up, they are left with a negative deficit. The coffee has transformed some of the essence stored in the kidneys into qi. This qi has been used, and now there is less stored essence. Since the blood and essence share a common source, coffee drinking may ultimately worsen any patterns associated with blood or kidney vacuities. Tea has a similar effect as coffee in that it transforms yin essence into yang qi and liberates that upward and outward through the body. However, the caffeine in black tea is usually only half as strong as in coffee.

Chocolate

Another problem food is chocolate. Chocolate is a combination of oil, sugar, and cocoa. We have seen that both oil and sugar are dampening and damaging to the spleen. Temporarily, the sugar will boost the spleen qi, but ultimately it will result in "sugar blues" or a hypoglycemic let down. Cocoa stirs the life gate fire. The life gate fire is another name for kidney yang or kidney fire, and kidney fire is the source of sexual energy and desire. It is said that chocolate is the food of love, and from the Chinese medical point of view, that is true. Since chocolate stimulates kidney fire at the same time as it temporarily boosts the spleen, it does give one rush of yang qi. In addition, this rush of yang qi does move depression and stagnation, at least short-term. So it makes sense that some people with liver depression, spleen vacuity, and kidney yang debility might crave chocolate. That being said, the sugar in chocolate ultimately damages the spleen, and the oil causes or worsens dampness.

Alcohol

Alcohol is both damp and hot according to Chinese medical theory. It strongly moves the qi and blood. Therefore, persons with liver depression qi stagnation will feel temporarily better from drinking alcohol. However, the sugar in alcohol damages the spleen and engenders dampness which "gums up the works," while the heat (yang) in alcohol can waste the blood (yin) and aggravate or inflame depressive liver heat. In particular, alcohol is contra-indicated in any kind of damp heat condition.

Hot, peppery foods

Spicy, peppery, "hot" foods also move the qi, thereby giving some temporary relief to liver depression qi stagnation. However, like alcohol, the heat in spicy hot foods wastes the blood and can inflame yang. Hot, peppery foods are specifically prohibited in damp heat patterns and conditions.

Sour foods

In Chinese medicine, the sour flavor is inherently astringing and constricting. Therefore, people with liver depression qi stagnation should be careful not to use vinegar and other intensely sour foods. Such sour flavored foods will only aggravate the qi stagnation by astringing and restricting the qi and blood all the more. This is also why sweet and sour foods, such as orange juice and tomatoes are particularly bad for people with liver depression and spleen vacuity. The sour flavor astringes and constricts the qi, while the sweet flavor damages the spleen and engenders dampness. So, whenever there is a problem with the free flow of the qi and blood, it is best to minimize or avoid excessively sour foods, such as vinegar.

Diet sodas

In my experience, diet sodas seem to contain something that damages the Chinese idea of the kidneys. They may not damage the spleen the same way that sugared sodas do, but that does not mean they are healthy and safe. I say that diet sodas damage the kidneys since a number of my patients over the years have reported that, when they drink numerous diet sodas, they experience terminal dribbling, urinary incontinence, and low back and knee soreness and weakness. When they stop drinking diet sodas, these symptoms disappear. Taken as a group, in Chinese medicine, these are kidney vacuity symptoms. Since the kidneys govern the bones and joints, it seems reasonable to avoid eating or drinking anything which causes the signs and symptoms of kidney weakness.

Foods which help nourish the blood

Qi & Wei

According to Chinese dietary therapy, all foods contain varying proportions of qi and *wei*. Qi means the ability to catalyze or promote yang function, while *wei* (literally meaning flavor) refers to a food's ability to nourish or construct yin substance. Since blood is relatively yin compared to qi being yang, a certain amount of food high in *wei* is necessary for a person to engender and transform blood. Foods which are high in *wei* as compared to qi are those which tend to be heavy, dense, greasy or oily, meaty or bloody. All animal products contain more *wei* than vegetable products. At the same time, black beans or, even better, black soybeans contain more *wei* than celery or lettuce.

When people suffer from joint pain due to blood vacuity failing to nourish the sinews or yin vacuity failing to strengthen the bones, they usually need to eat slightly more foods high in *wei*. This includes animal proteins and products, such as meat and eggs. It is said that flesh foods are very "compassionate" to the human

85

body. This word recognizes the fact that the animal's life has had to be sacrificed to produce this type of food. It also recognizes that, because such food is so close to the human body itself, it is especially nutritious. Therefore, when people suffer from vacuity rheumatic pain, eating some animal products usually is helpful and sometimes is down right necessary.

Animal foods vs. vegetarianism

Based on my many years of clinical experience, I have seen many Westerners adhering to a strict vegetarian diet develop, after several years, blood or yin vacuity patterns. This is especially the case in women who lose blood every month and must build babies out of the blood and yin essence. When women who are strict vegetarians come to me with various complaints, if they present the signs and symptoms of blood vacuity, such as a fat, pale tongue, pale face, pale nails, and pale lips, heart palpitations, insomnia, and fatigue with a fine, forceless pulse, I typically do recommend that they include a little animal food into their diet. In such cases, they commonly report to me how much better they feel imme-diately—how much more energy they have.

The downside of eating meat—besides the ethical issues—are that foods which are high in *wei* also tend to be harder to digest and to engender phlegm and dampness. Therefore, such foods should only be eaten in very small amounts at any one time. In addition, the weaker the person's spleen or the more phlegm and dampness they already have, the less such foods they should eat.

Remember above we said that the process of digestion first consisted of turning the food and drink ingested into 100° soup in the stomach. Therefore, soups and broths made out of animal flesh are the easiest and most digestible way of adding some animal-quality *wei* to a person's diet. When eating flesh itself, this should probably be limited to only one to two ounces per serving and only three or four such servings per week. According to Chinese dietary theory, the best foods for engendering and transforming blood and yin essence are organ meats and red or dark meats. This includes beef, buffalo, venison, lamb, and dark meat from chicken, turkey, goose, and duck. White meat fish and white meat fowl are less effective for building blood. However, white meat pork is also OK, as is ham.

One good recipe for adding more digestible *wei* to the diet of a person who is blood vacuous is to take a marrow bone and boil this with some cut vegetables, especially root vegetables, and black beans or black soybeans. Such a marrow bone, black bean, and vegetable soup is easy to digest and yet rich in *wei*.

Food allergies, leaky gut, candidiasis & parasites

Western research suggests that many patients with systemic rheumatic diseases, such as RA and SLE, suffer from various food allergies. Often these food allergies are due to "leaky gut syndrome." This means the intestinal walls are more permeable than they should be. Hence they allow large, undigested food molecules into the blood stream where they should not be and where they provoke allergic reactions. Often this type of leaky gut syndrome is due to or complicated by an overgrowth of yeast and fungi in the intestines. Everyone's intestines are home to many types of yeast and fungi. As long as their numbers stay in proportion to the protozoa and bacteria in the guts and as long as these fungi stay within the intestines themselves, no problem. However, when they overgrow, they often move out of the intestines and into the body. They do so by sending out shoots or buds which wiggle through the intestines, thus causing leaks in the intestinal walls. Once inside the body, these fungi eventually die, and, when they decompose, their foreign proteins also provoke allergic reactions.

If the body is constantly fighting off this and that foreign protein, eventually two things happen. First, the body no longer recognizes what it should and should not attack. Because the immune system loses its perspective due to being constantly overworked and revved up into high gear, the immune system may start attacking the body's own healthy tissue. This is called an autoimmune response, and RA and SLE are classified as autoimmune diseases. Secondly, because the immune system is so overworked, it may not adequately protect the body against true foreign proteins and pathogens. Thus the body is continually invaded and assaulted, causing the immune system to become even more dysfunctional. In such cases, it is not uncommon to find that other amoebas and protozoa which are regarded as parasites are able to establish themselves within the guts. This only makes the intestinal flora and fauna more "dysbiotic", meaning an unhealthy mix of intestinal populations, and hence the intestines function that much worse.

Food allergies, leaky gut syndrome, candidiasis, and parasites are mostly Western medical concepts. Nonetheless, the signs and symptoms of all these are described in Chinese medicine. In that case, they are mainly associated with spleen vacuity and dampness, damp heat, liver depression, and liver-kidney vacuities. Therefore, the anti-candida diet is essentially the same as the Chinese "clear, bland diet."

Some last words on diet

In conclusion, Western patients are always asking me what they should eat in order to cure their disease. However, when it comes to diet, sad to say, the issue is not so much what to eat as what not to eat. Diet most definitely plays a major role in the cause and perpetuation of many people's rheumatic complaints. Except in the case of vegetarians suffering from blood or yin vacuities, the issue is mainly what to avoid or minimize, not what to eat. Most of us know that coffee, chocolate, sugars and sweets, oils and fats, and alcohol are not good for us. Most of us know that we should be eating more complex carbohydrates and freshly cooked vegetables and less fatty meats. However, it's one thing to know these things and another to follow what we know.

To be perfectly honest, a clear bland diet *à la* Chinese medicine is not the most exciting diet in the world. It is the traditional diet of most lower and lower middle class peoples around the world living in temperate climates. It is the traditional diet of most of my readers' great grandparents. The point I am making here is that our modern Western diet which is high in oils and fats, high in sugars and sweets, high in animal proteins, and proportionally high in uncooked, chilled foods and drinks is a relatively recent aberration, and you can't fool Mother Nature.

When one switches to the clear, bland diet of Chinese medicine, at first one may suffer from cravings for more "flavorful" food. These cravings are, in many cases, actually associated with food "allergies." In other words, we may crave what is actually not good for us similar to a drunk's craving alcohol. After a few days, these cravings tend to disappear and we may be amazed that we don't miss some of our convenience or "comfort" foods as much as we thought we would. If one has been addicted to a food like sugar for many years, it does not take much to "fall off the wagon" and be addicted again. Therefore, perseverance is the key to long-term success. As the Chinese say, a million is made up of nothing but lots of ones, and a bucket is quickly filled by steady drips and drops.

Exercise

Exercise is the second of what are called the three free therapies. According to Chinese medicine, regular and adequate exercise has two basic benefits. First, exercise promotes the movement of the qi and quickening of the blood. Since all joint pain and rheumatic *bi* conditions by definition involve a lack of free flow, it is obvious that exercise is an important therapy for helping heal such *bi* conditions. Secondly, exercise benefits the spleen. The spleen's movement and transportation of the digestate is dependent upon the "qi mechanism." The qi mechanism describes the function of the qi in upbearing the pure and downbearing the turbid parts of digestion. For the qi mechanism to function properly, the qi must be flowing normally and freely. Since exercise moves and rectifies the qi, it also helps regulate and rectify the qi mechanism. This then results in the spleen's movement and transportation of foods and liquids and its subsequent engendering and transforming of the qi and blood. Because spleen vacuity typically complicate most chronic rheumatic complaints and because a healthy spleen checks and controls a depressed liver, exercise treats one of the other commonly encountered disease mechanisms in the majority of Westerner's suffering from stubborn joint pain. Therefore, it is easy to see that regular, adequate exercise is a vitally important component of any person's regime for either preventing or treating rheumatic complaints.

What kind of exercise is best?

In my experience, I find aerobic exercise to be the most beneficial for most people. By aerobic exercise, I mean *any* physical activity which raises one's heartbeat 80% above their normal resting rate and keeps it there for at least 20 minutes. To calculate your normal resting heart rate, place your fingers over the pulsing artery on the front side of your neck. Count the beats for 15 seconds and then multiply by four. This gives you your beats per minute or BPM. Now multiply your BPM by .8. Take the resulting number and add it to your resting BPM. This gives you your aerobic threshold of BPM. Next engage in any physical activity you like. After you have been exercising for five minutes, take your pulse for 15 seconds once again at the artery on the front side of your throat. Again multiply the resulting count by four and this tells you your current BPM. If this number is less than your aerobic threshold BPM, then you know you need to exercise harder or faster. Once you get your heart rate up to your aerobic threshold, then you need to keep exercising at the same level of intensity for at least 20 minutes. In order to insure that one is keeping their heartbeat high enough for long enough, one should recount their pulse every five minutes or so.

Depending on one's age and physical condition, different people will have to exercise harder to reach their aerobic threshold than others. For some, simply walking briskly will raise their heartbeat 80% above their resting rate. For others, they will need to do calisthenics, running, swimming, racquetball, or some other, more strenuous exercise. It really does not matter what the exercise is as long as it raises your heartbeat 80% above your resting rate and keeps it there for 20 minutes. However, there are two other criteria that should be met. One, the exercise should be something that is not too boring. If it is too boring, then you may have a hard time keeping up your schedule. Since most people do find aerobic exercises such as running, stationary bicycles, and stair-steppers boring, it is good to listen to music or watch TV in order to distract your mind from the tedium. Secondly, the type of exercise should not cause any damage to any parts of the body. For instance, running on pavement may cause knee problems for some people. Therefore, you should pick a type of exercise you enjoy but also one which will not cause any problems or worsen your pain. For patients with joint or soft tissue pain, swimming or water aerobics can be an effective way to get a good cardiovascular workout without any damage.

When doing aerobic exercise, it is best to exercise either every day or every other day. If one does do their aerobics at least once every 72 hours, then its cumulative effects will not be as great. Therefore, I recommend that most of my patients do some sort of aerobic exercises every day or every other day, three to four times per week *at least*. The good news is that there is no real need to exercise more than 30 minutes at any one time. Forty-five minutes per session is not going to be all that much better than 25 minutes per session. And 25 minutes four times per week is very much better than one hour once a week.

Precautions during exercise

When a person has joint pain, it is important that the type of exercise one gets does not further aggravate the injured or diseased joints. For instance, if one has *bi* pain in the knees, then running on a hard surface may actually make that pain worse. In that case, the pounding and stress of the running may only damage the tissues of the knees further, causing even more pain and inflammation which then retards the healing process. In that case, one will want to find some activity which either exercises those parts of the body which are not injured or which exercise the whole body without putting stress on the injured area. As stated above, for those with injuries of the lower extremities, exercising in water can still mobilize the qi and blood without the injured part bearing the weight and stress of the body in normal gravity. In that case, the buoyancy of the water helps offset earth's gravity, and one can mobilize the joints without causing further damage. In other words, even if one cannot exercise the injured or diseased joint itself, one can usually still find some kind of exercise which will get their qi and blood freely and smoothly flowing.

Deep relaxation

As we have seen above, rheumatic complaints are commonly associated with liver depression qi stagnation. Rheumatic *bi* and other types of joint pain keep us from doing what we want to do in our lives. In addition, the simple fact of pain is very stressful and irritating. Therefore, deep relaxation is the third of the three free therapies. For deep relaxation to be therapeutic medically, it needs to be more than just mental equilibrium. It needs to be somatic or bodily relaxation as well as mental repose. Most of us no longer recognize that every thought we think and feeling we feel is actually a felt physical sensation somewhere in our body. The words we use to describe emotions are all abstract nouns, such as anger, depression, sadness, and melancholy. However, in

Chinese medicine, *every emotion is associated with a change in the direction or flow of qi*. As we have said above, anger makes the qi move upward. Fear, on the other hand, makes the qi move downward. Therefore, anger "makes our gorge rise" or "blows our top", while fear may cause a "sinking feeling" or make us "pee in our pants." These colloquial expressions are all based on the age-old wisdom that all thoughts and emotions are not just mental but also bodily events. This is why it is not just enough to clear one's mind. Clearing one's mind is good, but for really marked therapeutic results, it is even better if one clears one's mind at the same time as relaxing every muscle in the body as well as the breath.

Guided deep relaxation tapes

The single most efficient and effective way for patients to practice such mental and physical deep relaxation is to do a daily, guided, progressive, deep relaxation audiotape. What I mean by guided is that a narrator on the tape leads one through the process of deep relaxation. Such tapes are progressive since they lead one through the body in a progressive manner, first relaxing one body part and then moving on to another. For instance, the narrator may say something to the effect that, as you exhale, you should feel your forehead get heavy and relaxed, softening and expanding, becoming warm and heavy. As you exhale again, now feel your cheeks get heavy and relaxed, softening and expanding, becoming warm and heavy. Breathe in and breathe out, letting your breath go without hindrance or hesitation. Breathing out, now feel your jaw muscles become heavy and relaxed, expanding and softening, becoming warm and heavy, etc., etc., throughout the entire body until one comes to the bottoms of one's feet.

There are innumerable such tapes on the market. These are usually sold in health food stores, New Age music and supply stores, or in bookstores with a good selection of New Age books. Over the years of suggesting this method of deep relaxation to my patients, I have found that each patient will have their own preferences in terms of the type of voice, male or female, the choice of words and imagery, whether there is background music or not, and the actual pace of the progression through the body, some narrators speaking a slightly different rate and rhythm. Therefore, I suggest listening to and even purchasing more than one such tape. One should find a tape which they like and can listen to without internal criticism or comment, going along like a cloud in the sky as the narrator's voice blows away all your mental and bodily stress and tension. If one has more than one tape, one can also switch every now and again from tape to tape so as not to become bored with the process or desensitized to the instructions.

Key things to look for in a good relaxation tape

In order to get the full therapeutic effect of such deep relaxation tapes, there are several key things to check for. First, be sure that the tape is a guided tape and not a subliminal relaxation tape. Subliminal tapes usually have music and any instructions to relax are given so quietly that they are not consciously heard. Although such tapes can help you feel relaxed when you do them, ultimately they do not teach you how to relax as a skill which can be consciously practiced and refined. Secondly, make sure the tape starts from the top of the body and works downward. Remember, anger makes the qi go upward in the body, and people with irritability and easy anger due to liver depression qi stagnation already have too much qi rising upward in their bodies. Such depressed qi typically needs not only to be moved but also downborne. Third, make sure the tape instructs you to relax your physical body. If you do not relax all your muscles or sinews, the qi cannot flow freely and the liver cannot be coursed. Depression is not resolved, and there will not be the same medically therapeutic effect. And lastly, be sure the tape instructs you to let your breath go with each exhalation. One of the symptoms of liver depression is a stuffy feeling in the chest which we then unconsciously try to relieve by sighing. Letting each exhalation go completely helps the lungs push the qi downward. This allows the lungs to control the liver at the same time as it downbears upwardly counterflowing angry liver qi.

The importance of daily practice

When I was an intern in Shanghai in the People's Republic of China, I was once taken on a field trip to a hospital clinic where they were using deep relaxation as a therapy with patients with high blood pressure, heart disease, stroke, migraines, and insomnia. The doctors at this clinic showed us various graphs plotting their research data on how such daily, progressive deep relaxation can regulate the blood pressure and body temperature and improve the appetite, digestion, elimination, sleep, energy, and mood. One of the things they said has stuck with me for 15 years: "Small results in 100 days, big results in 1,000." This means that if one does such daily, progressive deep relaxation *every single day for 100 days*, one will definitely experience certain results. What are these "small" results? These small results are improvements in all the parameters listed above: blood pressure, body temperature, appetite, digestion, elimination, sleep, energy, and mood. If these are "small" results, then what are the "big" results experienced in 1,000 days of practice? The "big" results are a change in how one reacts to stress—in other words, a change in one's very personality or character.

What these doctors in Shanghai stressed and what I have also experienced both personally and with my patients is that it is vitally important to do such daily, guided, progressive deep relaxation every single day, day in and day out for a solid three months at least and for a continuous three years at best. If one does such progressive, somatic deep relaxation every day, one will see every parameter or measurement of health and well-being improve. If one does this kind of deep relaxation only sporadically, missing a day here and there, it will feel good when you do it, but it will not have the marked, cumulative therapeutic effects it can. Therefore, perseverance is the real key to getting the benefits of deep relaxation.

The real test

Doing such a daily deep relaxation regime is like hitting tennis balls against a wall or hitting a bucket of balls at a driving range. It is only practice; it is not the real game itself. Doing a daily deep relaxation regime is not only in order to relieve one's immediate stress and strain. It is to learn a new skill, a new way to react to stress. The ultimate goal is to learn how to breathe out and immediately relax all one's muscles in the body in reaction to stress, rather than the common but unhealthy maladaption to stress of holding one's breath and tensing one's muscles. By doing such deep relaxation day after day, one learns how to relax any and every muscle in the body quickly and efficiently. Then, as soon as one recognizes they are feeling frustrated, stressed out, or uptight, they can immediately remedy those feelings at the same time as coursing their liver and rectifying their qi. This is the real test, the game of life. "Small results in 100 days, big results in 1,000."

Finding the time

If you're like me and most of my patients, you are probably asking yourself right now, "All this is well and good, but when am I supposed to find the time to eat well-balanced cooked meals, exercise at least every other day, and do a deep relaxation every day? I'm already stretched to the breaking point." I know. That's the problem.

As a clinician, I often wish I could wave a magic wand over my patients' heads and make them all healthy and well. I cannot. After close to two decades of working with thousands of patients, I know of no easy way to health. There is good living and there is easy living. Or perhaps I am stating this all wrong. What most people take as the easy way these days is to continue pushing their limits continually to the max. The so-called path of least resistance is actually the path of lots and lots of resistance. Unless you take time for yourself and find the time to eat well, exercise, and relax, no treatment is going to eliminate your rheumatic complaints completely. There is simply no pill you can pop or food you can eat that will get rid of the root causes of most chronic disease: poor diet, too little exercise, and too much stress. Even Chinese herbal medicine and acupuncture can only get their full effect if the diet and lifestyle is first adjusted. Sun Si-maio, the most famous Chinese doctor of the Tang dynasty (618-907 CE), who himself refused government office and lived to be 101, said: "First adjust the diet and lifestyle and only secondarily give herbs and acupuncture." Likewise, it is said today in China, "Three parts treatment, seven parts nursing." This means that any cure is only 30% due to medical treatment and 70% is due to nursing, meaning proper diet and lifestyle.

In my experience, this is absolutely true. Seventy percent of all disease will improve after three months of proper diet, exercise, relaxation, and lifestyle modification. Seventy percent! Each of us has certain nondiscretionary rituals we perform each day. For instance, you may always and without exception find the time to brush your teeth. Perhaps it is always finding the time to shower. For others, it may be always finding the time each day to eat lunch. And for 99.999% of us, we find time, no, we make the time to get dressed each day. The same applies to good eating, exercise, and deep relaxation. Where there's a will there's a way. If your joint pain and rheumatic complaints are bad enough, you can find the time to eat well, get proper exercise, and do a daily deep relaxation tape.

Conclusion

To get these benefits, one must make the necessary changes in eating and behavior. In addition, rheumatic complaints are not a condition that is cured once and forever like measles or mumps. When I say Chinese medicine can cure joint pain, I do not mean that you will never experience unwanted pain in your joints again. What I mean is that Chinese medicine can eliminate or

97

greatly reduce your symptoms *as long as you keep your diet and lifestyle together*. People being people, we all "fall off the wagon" from time to time and we all "choose our own poisons." I do not expect perfection from either my patients or myself. Therefore, I am not looking for a lifetime cure. Rather, I try to give my patients an understanding of what causes their disease and what they can do to minimize or eliminate its causes and mechanisms. It is then up to the patient to decide what is bearable and what is unbearable or what is an acceptable level of health. The Chinese doctor will have done their job when *you know how to correct your health to the level you find acceptable given the price you have to pay*.

Chinese Methods of Self-care for Rheumatic Complaints

In the previous chapters, we have seen how professionally practiced Chinese medicine treats joint pain, arthritis, and rheumatic complaints with acupuncture, moxibustion, and Chinese herbal medicine. These are all therapies which require a visit or visits to the office of a professional practitioner. Although acupuncture and Chinese medicine are the fastest growing professional alternative medicine in north America today, many North American communities are not currently served by a qualified local practitioner. However, one of the strong points of Chinese medicine is that it has consistently emphasized self-care. Therefore, within Chinese medicine, there are all sorts of treatments one can try in the comfort of your own home.

Below I have given a selection of such Chinese home remedies for joint pain and rheumatic complaints. If you choose to try any of these, start out slowly and cautiously and be sure to follow the directions. If you experience *any* negative side effects, stop and seek professional consultation. Chinese medicine when based on the correct pattern discrimination is without side effects. It heals by healing the entire person. Therefore, no side effects are expected or acceptable.

Qi gong

Qi means the qi we have been talking about repeatedly throughout this book. *Gong* means to discipline or train.

Therefore, *qi gong* exercises are exercises which train the qi. Although the words *qi gong* are no more than 100 years old, exercises for training the qi have been practiced in China since at least 500 BCE. In the People's Republic of China today, there is a renaissance of interest in *qi gong*, with *qi gong* classes, books, and research institutes sprouting up all over. Literally tens of millions of Chinese do some sort of *qi gong* every day. *Qi gong* can be done to promote health and prevent disease, while there are also *qi gong* exercises to treat almost every conceivable disease.

One simple *qi gong* exercise that anyone can do is to sit comfortably in a chair with your back straight. Breathing in, visualize the healing qi as a warm, milky light filling heaven above. Breathe this light in through the crown of your head as you inhale. Then as you exhale, visualize this light moving through your body to collect at the joint or joints which are affected. Imagine with each new breath that you are inhaling more and more healing qi from heaven. Then with each exhalation, wash the affected area in a bath of warm, healing qi and light. As you do this, feel the area become warm (as long as the condition is not a hot *bi*) and feel the qi moving to and through the affected area. Think that all pathogenic factors, such as wind, cold, dampness, stagnant qi, phlegm, and blood stasis are dissipated and that the area feels tingling with the effervescent feeling of flowing qi. One can continue like this from several minutes to a half hour or more. At the end of the session, visualize that the affected area is completely healed, think that it is pain free, and imagine that it is now ready to use again without limitation or disease.

If you suffer from hot *bi*, then feel this breath of life and light as a cool current bathing the affected area. Feel the congested heat dissipate and imagine that the swelling has dispersed.

To make this exercise even more powerful, you can pull the healing qi down from heaven with your hands on each inhalation, and then direct it to the affected joint or body part with the hands on the exhalation, thus mobilizing the qi even more by coordinating the mind, breath, and the movement of the body.

Other simple yet profoundly effective *qi gong* exercises for arthritis and rheumatic complaints can be found in Dr. Yang Jingming's excellent book, *Qigong for Arthritis*. Other titles of good *qi gong* books and videotapes are given in the annotated bibliography in the back of this book.

Chinese self-massage

Massage has always been a very important part of Chinese medicine. Rubbing, kneading, tapping, and pinching the body are all ways of stimulating the flow of qi through the channels and vessels. Since rheumatic *bi* conditions are, by definition, problems associated with a lack of free flow, it stands to reason that self-massage would be a good way to help treat this condition.

Fan Ya-li, a professor of Chinese medical massage, previously affiliated with the Shandong College of Chinese Medicine and now working in the United States, has written a book on Chinese self-massage titled, *Chinese Self-massage Therapy: The Easy Way to Health*, also published by Blue Poppy Press. The entire last section of this book is devoted to self-massage regimes for various types of joint pain. These include stiff neck and cervical arthritis, periarthritis of the shoulder, tennis elbow, carpal tunnel syndrome, acute lumbar sprain, chronic lumbar pain, and knee joint pain. Although we cannot reprint the entire section from Dr. Fan's book, the following Chinese self-massage regime for the treatment of periarthritis of the shoulder gives a good idea of what Chinese self-massage is like.

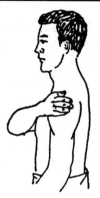

Begin by kneading the shoulder with the heel of the palm of the opposite hand. Knead every side of the affected shoulder, beginning with weak pressure and gradually applying stronger pressure. Do this for 3-5 minutes.

Next, pinch and grasp the muscles of the affected shoulder with the thumb, index, and middle fingers of the other hand. Pinch and grasp all around the shoulder for 3-5 minutes, grasping more on the deltoid muscle on the side of the shoulder.

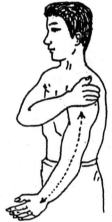

Now pinch and grasp the upper arm with the thumb, index, and middle finger of the other hand. Pinch and grasp the muscles on the front and back of the affected upper arm from the shoulder to the elbow 30-50 times.

This should be followed by pressing and kneading any particularly tender points around the affected shoulder, beginning with weak pressure and gradually pressing more and more strongly. At the same time, mobilize the shoulder. Do this for 2-3 minutes.

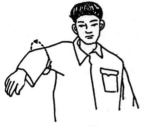

Rotate the affected shoulder joint in both directions approximately 10 times. Begin with small circles and increase to large circles.

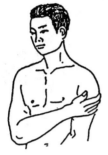

And finally, rub the shoulder and upper arm with the palm of the opposite hand, rubbing every side of the shoulder and upper arm until the whole area feels warm to the touch.

Now bend at the waist, stretch out the arm, and rotate the shoulder. The movement should start small and then gradually get larger. Likewise, the movement should start slowly and then gradually pick up speed.

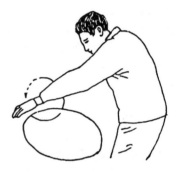

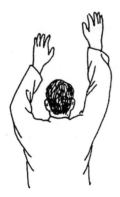

Stand facing a wall. With either both or only one hand, raise the arms as high as possible as if you were climbing the wall. Repeat this several times, increasing the height each time if possible.

This regime is almost over when you bring both hands behind the body. With the healthy hand holding the wrist of the affected shoulder, lead the affected arm backward as far as possible. Do this repeatedly for several times.

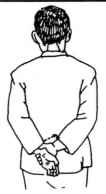

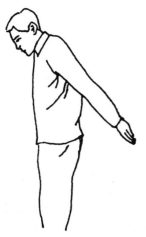

And finish up by swinging either both or only the affected arm backward and forward in an arc, making sure that the arm is very heavy and loose. By the time you finish, the shoulder should feel less stiff and painful and the whole arm should feel heavy, relaxed, tingling, warm, and full of free-flowing qi.

Although a single self-massage treatment should make the affected joint or area feel better, self-massage is most effective when done on a regular basis every day for a number of days in a row. In this sense, the effects of Chinese self-massage are cumulative. Therefore, perseverance is the key to getting good results with Chinese self-massage as it is with most of the self-help techniques suggested in this chapter.

Magnet therapy

The Chinese have used magnet therapy since at least the Tang dynasty (618-907 CE). Placing magnets on the body is a safe and painless way of stimulating acupuncture points without inserting needles through the skin. Since magnets can be taped onto points and "worn" for days at a time, Chinese magnet therapy is able to provide easy, low cost, continuous treatment. It is also possible to tape on magnets at night and to wear them to bed. Special adhesive magnets for stimulating acupuncture points, such as Accu-Band Magnets, Corimag, or Epaule Patch TDK Magnets, may be purchased from:

Oriental Medical Supply Co.
1950 Washington St.
Braintree, MA 02184
Tel: (617) 331-3370 or 800-323-1839
Fax: (617) 335-5779

These magnets range in strength from 400-9,000 gauss, the unit measuring magnetic strength. For the treatments below, one can try 400-800 gauss magnets.

The easiest way of using body magnets to free the flow of qi and blood in painful joints is to place a magnet with its south pole downward on top of the skin directly over the most painful spots. The more accurately one can locate these points, the better will be the result. In this case, there are two types of painful spots. The first is the most painful place when one moves the joint, while the second is found by pressing with the fingertips all around the soft tissue surrounding the point. Points which are painful to palpation are called *a shi* points in China. This is because Chinese will say, "*a shi!*" ("That's it!") when the point is pressed.

Remember that all pain is a symptom of the lack of free flow of the qi and blood. Most rheumatic *bi* pain is due to either wind, cold, dampness, heat, phlegm, or blood stasis hindering and obstructing the free flow of qi. According to Chinese medical theory, these are all types of repletion. This means that they are something extra which should not be there. The principle for treating such "repletions" in Chinese medicine is to drain them. The south side of a magnet is the draining side, while the north side is the supplementing side. If you first try the south side down on any *a*

105

shi points and this makes the pain worse, try flipping the magnet over and put the north side down.

If the pain is vacuous in nature, meaning that it is worse after inactivity, at the end of the day, or when fatigued, the lack of free flow may not be due to anything blocking the channels and network vessels. Rather, it may be due to a simple lack of qi and blood to nourish and insure the proper function of the sinews and vessels. In that case, put the north side of the magnet down. However, in such "vacuity" conditions, it is usually harder to find actual tender spots.

One can get more sophisticated with the use of north and south magnets for the treatment of rheumatic complaints if one knows the locations of certain acupoints and the courses of the major channels. In that case, one can promote the free flow of qi and blood by placing a south magnet skin downward on a point "below" the affected joint and a north side facing magnet skin down on a point "above" the affected joint. Below and above here do not mean what they normally do. Each channel travels in a certain direction. Above means above the affected joint or area on the side the qi is coming from. Below means below the affected area on the side of the joint to which the qi is flowing. In this case, the south side down magnet stimulates the dispersing movement of accumulated qi, while the north side magnet attracts that moving qi to move towards it. Since most lay readers will not know the locations of the points, the courses of the channels, nor the directions of their flow, one can visit a local acupuncturist who can give you a short course in these matters specific to the joint you are attempting to treat.

Seven star hammer

A seven star hammer is a small hammer or mallet with seven small needles embedded in its head. Nowadays in China, it is often called a skin or dermal needle and is also available in a single-use disposable version. It is one of the ways a person can stimulate various acupuncture points without actually inserting a needle into the body. Seven star hammers can be used either for people who are afraid of regular acupuncture, for children, or for those who wish to treat their condition at home. When the points to be stimulated are on the front of the body, this technique can be done by oneself. When they are located on the back of the body, this technique can be done by a family member or friend. This is a very easy technique which does not require any special training or expertise.

When treating joint pain with a seven star hammer, first wipe the affected area with rubbing alcohol or hydrogen peroxide to disinfect the skin. Then lightly tap all around the affected joint. If the condition is due to wind, cold, and/or dampness, use medium strength and do not tap so hard as to cause any bleeding. The skin should simply become red in color all around the affected joint or area. This redness is due to increased blood flow in this area. Since the qi is what moves the blood, seven star hammering like this stimulates the flow of both qi and blood.

If the condition is associated with blood stasis, damp heat, or heat *bi*, then I do recommend tapping hard enough to cause not only redness of the skin but also a little light bleeding. Such bleeding helps drain static blood and/or pathogenic heat at the same time as it increases the flow of qi and blood locally. To avoid any possibility of infection, be sure to carefully disinfect the area after treatment, especially if you have caused any bleeding.

If there is lack of flow due to insufficiency of the qi and blood, then only tap very softly. This will help stimulate the qi and blood to move to and hence supplement and nourish the affected area. The basic rule of thumb with seven star hammering is that light tapping is supplementing, while heavy tapping is draining. The heavier the tapping the more draining this technique is.

Seven star hammering can be done on any individual joint in the body. It may also be done on top of and on either side of the spine. If there is neck joint pain, then one can tap all along the spine in the neck and the strap muscles to either side. Likewise, if there is low back pain, one can tap on top of the spine and on the long muscles to either side all up and down the affected area. This can be done either once or twice per day. Since this is not a very strong method of stimulation, like self-massage, it needs to be done consistently every day for a number of days in a row in order to see marked results.

Seven star hammers can be purchased through the mail from Oriental Medical Supply Co. whose address and telephone ordering numbers are given on page 105. After each treatment, the hammer should be soaked in rubbing alcohol or hydrogen peroxide in order to disinfect it between uses. Since these hammers are very inexpensive, I recommend that each person have their own and not share them with others. Since you may cause a little bleeding doing this technique, you do not want to risk any cross-infection between persons sharing a single hammer. Slightly more expensive versions of these hammers are available made out of surgical steel. These can be boiled or cooked in a pressure cooker for 30 minutes to help sterilize them. Plastic versions can only be soaked in a disinfectant solution. Single-use disposable type "hammers" are thrown away after each treatment.

Thread moxibustion

Thread moxibustion refers to burning extremely tiny cones or "threads" of aged Oriental mugwort (Folium Artemisiae Argyii, *Ai Ye*) directly on top of certain acupuncture points. When done correctly, this is a very simple and effective way of strongly stimulating the flow of qi and blood and adding yang qi to the body without causing a burn or scar.

To do thread moxa, one must first purchase the finest grade of Japanese moxa wool. This is available from Oriental Medical Supply Co. mentioned above. It is listed in their catalog under the name Gold Direct Moxa. Pinch off a very small amount of this loose moxa wool and roll it lightly between the thumb and forefingér. What you want to wind up with is a very loose, very thin thread of moxa smaller than a grain of rice. It is important that this thread not be too large or too tightly wrapped.

Next, rub a very thin film of Tiger Balm or Temple of Heaven Balm on the point to be moxaed. These are camphored Chinese medical salves which are widely available in North American health food stores. Be sure to apply nothing more than the thinnest film of salve. If such a Chinese medicated salve is not available, then wipe the point with a *tiny* amount of vegetable oil. Stand the thread of moxa up perpendicularly directly over the point to be moxaed. The oil or balm should provide enough stickiness to make the thread stand on end. Light the tread with a burning incense stick. As the thread burns down towards the skin, you will feel more and more heat. Immediately remove the burning thread when you begin to feel the burning thread go from hot to too hot. *Do not burn yourself.* It is better to pull the thread off too soon than too late. In this case, more is not better than enough. (If you do burn yourself, apply some *Ching Wan Hong* ointment. This is a Chinese burn salve which is available at Chinese apothecaries and is truly wonderful for treating all sorts of burns. It should be in every home's medicine cabinet.)

Having removed the burning thread and extinguished it between your two fingers, repeat this process again. To make this process go faster and more efficiently, one can roll a number of threads before starting the treatment. Each time the thread burns down close to the skin, pinch it off the skin and extinguish it *before* it starts to burn you. If you do this correctly, your skin will get red and hot to the touch but you will not raise a blister. Because everyone's skin is different, the first time you do this, only start out with three or four threads. Each day, increase this number until you reach nine to twelve threads per treatment.

This technique can be used either to treat local areas of stubborn pain or it can be used to supplement a vacuous and weak spleen and kidneys. When localized joint pain is particularly recalcitrant (*i.e.*, stubborn) to treatment, thread moxibustion is one of the best techniques within Chinese medicine. Often, thread moxibustion can relieve pain that insertion of acupuncture needles, cupping, or other methods cannot. Like magnet therapy discussed above, one should find the tenderest, most painful spot. The more accurately you locate such spots, the more effective this treatment will be. These spots may be either places which are painful when the joint is mobilized or places which are extremely sensitive to pressure when pushed with the fingertips. In either case, burn five to seven threads of moxa directly over such spots and increase this number of threads up to 10-12 per day. Do this every day for a number of days in a row. Continue for several days even after all the pain has disappeared in order to consolidate the treatment effect.

Many patients with chronic rheumatic *bi* conditions, and especially those with systemic autoimmune diseases, exhibit spleen and possibly also kidney vacuity patterns. In such cases, local treatment is not enough. Until or unless the spleen is fortified and the kidneys are warmed and invigorated, local treatment will not produce completely satisfactory or stable results. Happily, there are three points which are easy to locate and can be thread moxaed in order to supplement the spleen and kidneys. These are:

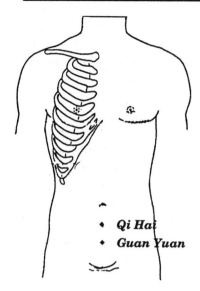

Qi Hai (Conception Vessel 6): This point is located two finger-breadths below the navel on the midline of the lower abdomen. This point supplements the qi of the entire body.

Guan Yuan (Conception Vessel 4): This point is located four finger-breadths below the navel on the midline of the lower abdomen. This points especially supplements the yang qi and essence of the kidneys.

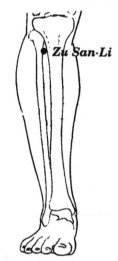

Zu San Li (Stomach 36): This point is located three finger-breadths below the lower, outer corner of the kneecap in a depression between the muscles on the lateral side of the lower leg. This point supplements the engenderment and transformation of the qi and blood of the entire body via the spleen and stomach.

Although these points are quite easy to locate, I recommend visiting a local professional acupuncturist so that they can teach you how to do this technique safely and effectively and to show you how to locate these three points accurately.

In Chinese medicine, this technique is considered a longevity and health preservation technique. It is great for those people whose yang qi has already begun to decline due to the inevitable aging process. It should also always be done starting from the topmost

111

point and moving downward. This is so as not to lead heat to counterflow upward. If there is any doubt about whether this technique is appropriate for you, please see a professional practitioner for a diagnosis and individualized recommendation.

Pole moxibustion

Pole moxibustion is another way of using aged Oriental mugwort (Folium Artemisiae Argyii, *Ai Ye*) to increase the flow of qi and blood in the treatment of arthritis or rheumatic complaints. In this case the moxa *does not touch the skin* but is held over or under specific acupuncture points or areas of pain. This method is especially effective in cases of yang vacuity cold pain where the discomfort is clearly improved by warmth. There may also be other symptoms of vacuity cold such as cold feet or legs, abdominal pain which is improved by warmth, excessive urination, a pale or bluish tongue, or a slow, deep pulse.

To use this method of moxibustion, one needs to light the moxa pole or stick and hold it over or under the affected areas of pain for several minutes until the skin has turned quite pink, usually five-seven minutes. Be careful not to burn the skin. When the heat feels scorching, move the stick away for a few seconds and then back again. One can use a chicken-pecking motion repeatedly moving the stick closer to the skin and then farther away or use a circular motion going around and around the area to be treated. This can be done at any joint, although it should not be administered over the heart, on the face, over the external genitalia, or on the center of the back just behind the heart.

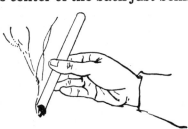

There are two types of moxa poles. One type makes smoke, the other doesn't. Both are available from Oriental Medical Supply Co. listed above or from a local acupuncture practitioner. If you have a negative reaction to smoke, the smokeless version can be used. However, in Chinese medicine, it is thought that the smoke itself has therapeutic value and will increase the effectiveness of the treatment.

Pole moxa can be used every day or every other day. If you are unsure about these instructions, a local acupuncture practitioner can instruct you in the correct use of this type of therapy. As with any of these suggestions, if the use of moxa seems to be making your symptoms worse, discontinue immediately and see a local practitioner to clarify your diagnosis.

Hydrotherapy

Hydrotherapy means water therapy and is also a part of traditional Chinese medicine. There are several different water treatments for helping relieve joint pain and rheumatic complaints. If dampness is the major obstructing factor in your rheumatic compliant, then you probably will not choose hydrotherapy as a major part of your healing regime. However, if wind, cold, or heat are the major factors, then you can use hydrotherapy safely and effectively. It is also possible to use hydrotherapy if dampness is only a contributory or secondary factor.

As we have seen above, heat is yang and yang is associated with movement and transformation. When the body obtains warmth, the qi and blood flow more freely and easily. Although Western medicine, looking inside the body microscopically, says that the tissues are inflamed in most rheumatic complaints, that does not mean applying ice is really a good idea. The Chinese doctor does not look inside the joint. Rather, we infer what is going on inside by what manifests on the outside. Unless there is redness and heat on the outside of the body, we are probably going to

113

recommend warm applications rather than cold. Cold is yin and, therefore, is associated with stillness and contraction. When the body obtains cold, that cold inhibits and congeals the flow of qi and blood. Since pain implies lack of free flow already, except in cases of very recent traumatic injury with marked redness and heat or cases of hot *bi*, Chinese doctors always choose warm water applications for the treatment of rheumatic complaints.

Therefore, for acute joint pain due to wind, cold, or damp *bi*, one should heat some water and soak a cotton towel in it. Wring it out and apply to the affected area. The towel should be as hot as possible without burning the body. Cover with another dry towel and keep in place for 15 minutes. Do this once every hour. After removing this hot compress, rub some very cold water over the surface briefly in order to close the pores. This will keep any further external excesses from invading and settling in the affected area. Then cover the body and be sure not to get chilled.

For acute joint pain due to heat *bi* or damp heat *bi*, dip a cotton cloth in cold water and wrap loosely around the affected area. Pin this in place but be sure that the cloth is loose. Do not make the cloth so tight it constricts the joint and cuts off the flow of qi and blood. We want the qi and blood to flow through the area as freely as possible. However, we also need to clear the heat. In order to clear heat and reduce inflammation, sprinkle some cold water on the cloth every 15 minutes or so to keep the compress continuously cold.

For chronic joint pain, warm water soaks, hot baths, or hot steam baths are recommended. Generally, one should continue the hot water treatment for at least 20 minutes at a time. However, one should not stay in the hot water or steam bath for more than a maximum of two hours at any given time. As with acute joint pain, warm water applications for chronic rheumatic complaints should be followed by a very brief application of cold water in order to close the pores. Similarly, one must bundle up and stay warm afterwards so as to avoid further invasion.

114

For chronic joint pain it is also possible to spray the affected area with hot water for several minutes. The more pressure the better. Many modern shower heads allow for a focused stream of water under some pressure. Then switch to 15 seconds of intensely cold water. Alternate back and forth like this several times, always using the hot water for a long time and the cold water for a very short duration, always beginning with warm water and finishing with a very short application of cold.

Chinese patent medicines

There are a number of ready-made Chinese herbal medicines which are available over the counter in Chinese apothecaries and a growing number of health food stores around the United States and Canada. These are commonly Chinese patent medicines. Although it is best to get an individualized pattern discrimination from a qualified professional practitioner of Chinese medicine who can then write you your own, individually crafted Chinese herbal formula, if such a practitioner is not available, then one can experiment a little on their own. However, please remember that Chinese herbal medicine is prescribed for patterns of imbalance, not diseases, even notwithstanding what is often written in English on such patent medicines' labels.

Du Huo Ji Sheng Wan (Du Huo & Loranthus Pills)

These pills are also for chronic, enduring wind, cold, damp *bi* accompanied by a qi and blood or liver-kidney vacuity. This means that these pills are not appropriate for damp heat or heat *bi* and should also not be taken unless there are a collection of kidney vacuity signs and symptoms listed above. All the ingredients in this formula are vegetable in origin. The recommended dosage is nine pills, two times per day.

Feng Shi Xiao Tong Wan, also spelled *Feng Shih Hsiao Tung Wan* (Wind Dampness Dispersing Pain Pills)

These pills primarily treat wind damp *bi* mixed with blood stasis. Blood stasis is evidenced by fixed, sharp pain, severe pain, stubborn pain, and pain which is worse at night in patients with engorged or varicose veins, purplish tongue, a history of traumatic injury to the affected area, women with menstrual pain, uterine fibroids, endometriosis, or ovarian cysts, the elderly in general, or lots of "liver" or "age" spots.

Guan Jie Yan Wan (Close Down Joint Inflammation Pills)

These pills treat wind, cold, damp *bi*. Because one of their ingredients is Ephedra (Herba Ephedrae, *Ma Huang*), these pills are best if there is a recent onset, exterior pattern. Because Ephedra very powerfully resolves the exterior and "out thrusts" yang qi, its long-term or excessive usage can lead to yin vacuity and qi vacuity. Therefore, these pills should only be used short-term and by persons not suffering from simultaneous yin vacuity. If you try these pills and they make you feel "hyper", jumpy, jittery, anxious, or cause pounding in your heart, *stop taking them immediately* and seek a consultation from a qualified professional practitioner. Although these pills can be very effective for some people, they can cause side effects if taken by a person with the wrong pattern. The recommended dosage is eight pills, three times per day.

Feng Shi Pian, also erroneously labeled *Hong She Wan* (Wind Damp Tablets)

These pills are for wind, damp, cold *bi* primarily in the lower part of the body and complicated by low back pain. They also contain Ephedra and so the same cautions apply to these as to the pills above. The recommended dosage is two pills one time per day.

116

San She Dan Zhui Feng Wan, also spelled *San She Tan Chui Feng Wan* (Three Snake Gallbladder Expel Wind Pills)

These pills are for stubborn *bi* conditions complicated by blood stasis entering the network vessels and phlegm obstruction. If stasis endures for a long time, it is said to enter the network vessels. These are the myriad tiny vessels which criss-cross the body similar to the capillaries of Western medicine. If the blood becomes static in these tiny network vessels, special medicinals are necessary to enter these network vessels and free their flow. In addition, enduring blood stasis is also often complicated by phlegm obstruction since the blood and body fluids flow together and "share a common source." The recommended dose is 10 pills each time, two times per day.

Te Xiao Yao Tong Ling (Specially Effective Low Back Remedy), also called Specific Lumbaglin

These pills are designed to treat low back pain due to liver blood-kidney yin and yang vacuity complicated by blood stasis. This usually means chronic low back pain in a somewhat older person. The recommended dosage is one-two capsules three times per day.

Du Zhong Feng Shi Wan, also spelled *Tu Zhing Feng Shi Wan* (Eucommia Wind Dampness Pills)

These pills treat wind, damp, cold *bi* primarily of the low back or complicated by liver-kidney vacuity weakness. The recommended dosage is four-six pills two times per day.

Xiao Huo Luo Dan (Small Quicken the Network Vessels Elixir)

These pills are very hot in nature. Therefore, they are specifically for cold *bi* possibly complicated by phlegm and blood stasis. The recommended dosage is six pills, two-three times per day.

Ge Jie Da Bu Wan (Gecko Greatly Supplementing Pills)

These pills supplement the qi and blood, yin and yang. In addition, they include ingredients to strengthen the sinews and the bones. They work best for low back and lower extremity pain due to vacuity as opposed to *bi*. The recommended dosage is three-five capsules, three times per day.

Tian Qi Du Zhong Wan, also spelled *Ting Zat Do Zhung Wan* (Notoginseng & Eucommia Pills)

These pills are for the treatment of chronic *bi*, primarily in the elderly. The *bi* is cold impediment and the condition is complicated by both kidney vacuity and blood stasis. The recommended dosage is five pills four times per day.

These are only some of the commonly available Chinese patent medicines for the treatment of *bi* conditions and joint pain. Self-medication is never the wisest choice. Chinese herbal medicine is not safe because it is herbal. Many of the ingredients in these pills are not inherently safe. They are only safe at the proper dosage in the proper pattern. Therefore, my best advice is to seek an individually written Chinese herbal prescription from a qualified professional practitioner. On no account should you take Chinese herbal pills, sometimes sold under the name Black Pearls, which do not come in a box, are unlabeled, and without a list of the ingredients. Some Chinese companies do unscrupulously manufacture combinations of Chinese herbs and Western prescription medications which are left unlabeled on the packaging. Although these pills can provide seemingly miraculous symptomatic relief, they can also cause all the same side effects as corticosteroids. *Do not take these!* The patent medicines listed above are, to the best of my knowledge, unadulterated by Western drugs and are safe to take when matched with the proper Chinese pattern and in the correct dosage.

Some other pills for arthritis pain list tiger bone as one of their ingredients. While chemical analysis reveals that most of these products do not actually include any tiger bone, it is my belief that even *suggesting* the use of tiger bone in any product contributes to the endangerment and possible extinction of tigers worldwide. Therefore, products which list this as one of their ingredients are not included here.

Chinese herbal wines

In Chinese medicine, alcohol is said to quicken the healing effects of other medicinals as well as being especially effective for moving the qi and quickening the blood. Although many people with systemic rheumatic complaints, such as RA and SLE should not drink alcohol, there are a number of Chinese medicinal wines which can help relieve various types of *bi* conditions. A number of these "rheumatism wines" are available in pharmacies and liquor stores in Chinatowns in north America. However, they can also be easily made in one's own home.

Below are a selection of Chinese medicinal wines for rheumatic *bi* conditions which you can make yourself. Because alcohol is by nature hot, these medicinal wines are best for wind, damp, cold *bi*. They are also best taken during the winter when the weather is cold. In China, it is mostly older people who use such medicinal wines, people whose life gate fire has begun to decline and their qi and blood are no longer moving freely and easily. For more information about such Chinese medicinal wines, see Bob Flaws's book *Chinese Medicinal Wines & Elixirs* also published by Blue Poppy Press.

Du Huo Shen Fu Jiu (Angelica Pubescens, Codonopsis & Aconite Wine)

This wine scatters cold and dispels dampness, warms the middle and stops pain. It is meant for the treatment of low back and

119

lower leg swelling and pain in a person whose body is constitutionally weak. To make this wine, take Radix Angelicae Pubescentis (*Du Huo*), 35g, Radix Lateralis Praeparatus Aconiti Carmichaeli (*Fu Zi*), 35g, and Radix Codonopsitis Pilosulae (*Dang Shen*), 20g. Grind these three ingredients into a fine powder in a coffee grinder and place in a large jar. Soak in one quart of alcohol, such as vodka or brandy, and allow to tincture for five-seven days. Drink this daily when one feels cold or one feels pain. Only take this wine if your feet are constantly cold, if your pain is worsened by exposure to cold and improved by exposure to warmth, and if you have no signs or symptoms of heat.

Dang Gui Song Ye Jiu (Angelica Sinensis & Pine Needles Wine)

This wine scatters wind, dispels cold, and quickens the blood. It is indicated for wind cold *bi* complicated by blood stasis. It is made by taking two big handfuls of fresh pine needles and Radix Angelicae Sinensis (*Dang Gui*), 150g. Put these ingredients in one quart or liter of brandy or vodka and allow to steep for six-seven weeks. At the end of that time, remove the dregs and reserve the liquid. Drink this medicinal wine when you feel the pain.

Hei Dou Qiang Huo Jiu (Black Soybean & Notopterygium Wine)

This wine resolves the exterior and tracks down wind, overcomes dampness and stops pain. It is indicated for wind damp *bi* possibly complicated by blood vacuity not nourishing the sinews. Thus there is joint pain and especially stiffness accompanied by a pale face, pale lips, pale nails, pale tongue, dry skin, and dry hair. The ingredients in this wine are Radix Et Rhizoma Notopterygii (*Qiang Huo*), 15g, Radix Ledebouriellae Divaricatae (*Fang Feng*), 10g, and dry fried black soybeans (*Hei Dou*), 30g. Grind the above three ingredients into powder in a coffee grinder and soak in 200ml of rice wine or sake. Allow to soak for one week and then drink a small amount each evening either before or after dinner.

Pai Jiu Jiu (Expel Wind Wine)

This wine courses wind, scatters cold, and dispels dampness. It can be used to treat wind, damp, cold *bi* conditions. It is made by taking Radix Ledebouriellae Divaricatae (*Fang Feng*), 30g, Rhizoma Cimicifugae (*Sheng Ma*), 30g, Cortex Cinnamomi Cassiae (*Rou Gui*), 30g, Radix Lateralis Praeparatus Aconiti Carmichaeli (*Fu Zi*), 30g, Radix Angelicae Pubescentis (*Du Huo*), 30g, and Radix Et Rhizoma Notopterygii (*Qiang Huo*), 30g, grind these into powder, and soak for five-seven days in a liter or quart of brandy or vodka. Take 20ml each time, two times per day.

Dan Shen Du Zhong Jiu (Salvia & Eucommia Wine)

This wine quickens the blood and opens the network vessels, nourishes the liver and supplements the kidneys. It is used to treat blood stasis with simultaneous liver blood, and kidney yin and/or yang vacuity. Mostly this manifests as chronic low back and lower extremity pain in older patients. Its ingredients are Cortex Eucommiae Ulmoidis (*Du Zhong*), 60g, Radix Salviae Miltiorrhizae (*Dan Shen*), 60g, and Radix Ligustici Wallichii (*Chuan Xiong*), 40g. Grind these into powder and place in a large jar. Cover with one liter or quart of vodka or brandy and allow to soak for five-seven days. Then remove the dregs and drink a small amount every evening either before or after dinner.

Ling Pi Di Huang Jiu (Epimedium & Rehmannia Wine)

This wine supplements the kidneys and invigorates yang, dispels wind and dampness, and strengthens the sinews and bones. It treats lack of strength and pain of the low back and chronic wind damp *bi* in patients with a vacuous constitution or in the elderly. Its ingredients are Herba Epimedii (*Xian Ling Pi*), 250g, and cooked Radix Rehmanniae (*Shu Di*), 150g. Grind the above two ingredients and soak them for 5-7 days in two liters of vodka or brandy. Drink some of this each evening either before or after dinner.

If one likes their alcohol a little sweeter, then use brandy as the tincturing agent. If one likes their alcohol drier, then use vodka. If one does not like or cannot stand strong spirits, then use sake or rice wine.

Chinese herbal teas

When a professional practitioner writes an individualized prescription, the medicinals are usually taken as a decoction. This means that four to twenty or more Chinese medicinals are placed in water and boiled for thirty minutes to more than one hour. This results in a very strong medicinal soup which most Westerners would hardly relate to as a tea. However, in Chinese medicine, there are simpler drinks made with only one or two ingredients which are actually drunk as a tea and are sometimes made with tea (Folium Camilliae Theae, *Cha Ye*). A number of these can be used as home remedies for rheumatic *bi* complaints.

Jiang Can Liang Jiang Cha (Bombyx & Alpinia Tea)

This tea scatters cold, dispels wind, and stops pain. It can be used to treat wind, cold, damp *bi* pain. Its ingredients are equal amounts of Bombyx Batriticatus (*Jiang Can*), Rhizoma Alpiniae Officinari (*Gao Liang Jiang*), and green tea. Grind these three ingredients into fine powder and store in a dry place. To use, take 3 grams of this powder and steep in a cup of boiling water. This tea can be drunk two-three times per day.

Du Huo Cha (Angelica Pubescens Tea)

This tea is made from a single ingredient, Radix Angelicae Pubescentis (*Du Huo*). Boil 20g of this herb in water, remove the dregs, and drink freely throughout the day as tea. It dispels wind, scatters cold, and disinhibits dampness. It is used to treat wind, damp, cold *bi* pain in the joints, especially if this pain wanders about from joint to joint.

122

Mu Gua Cha (Chinese Quince Tea)

This tea soothes the sinews and quickens the network vessels, harmonizes the stomach and transforms dampness. It can be used for bone and joint pain primarily due to damp *bi* and primarily in the lower part of the body. It is made by taking Fructus Chaenomelis Lagenariae (*Mu Gua*), 15-20g, Cortex Radicis Acanthopanacis (*Wu Jia Pi*), 12g, and honey mix-fried Radix Glycyrrhizae (*Zhi Gan Cao*), 6g, and boiling these in 500ml of water for 15 minutes. Drink one packet of this tea per day. You can reboil the herbs in order to make more liquid if necessary.

Yi Mi Fang Feng Cha (Coix & Ledebouriella Tea)

This tea dispels wind and eliminates dampness. It treats heaviness, swelling, and soreness due to damp *bi*. It consists of Semen Coicis Lachryma-jobi (*Yi Yi Ren*), 30g, and Radix Ledebouriellae Divaricatae (*Fang Feng*), 10g. Boil these two medicinals in water and drink as a tea, one packet per day. This tea is also suitable if there is a slight amount of heat as well as dampness as evidenced by slight redness and slight heat in the affected joint.

Gu Sui Bu Cha (Drynaria Tea)

This tea is made out of Rhizoma Drynariae (*Gu Sui Bu*), 50g, and Ramulus Cinnamomi Cassiae (*Gui Zhi*), 15g. These are boiled in water and the resulting beverage drunk warm throughout the day. Use one packet each day. This tea quickens the blood and scatters cold, supplements the kidneys and strengthens the low back. It can be used to treat low back sprain as well as chronic low back pain due to kidney vacuity and/or blood stasis.

For more information on Chinese medicinal teas and an even wider selection of teas for treating rheumatic complaints, see Zong Xiao-fan and Gary Liscum's *Chinese Medicinal Teas: Simple,*

Proven Folk Formulas for Common Diseases & Promoting Health also published by Blue Poppy Press.

Chinese herbal porridges

Similar to Chinese medicinal wine and teas, there is a whole repertoire of medicinal porridges within Chinese medicine. Sometimes called congee, these medicinal porridges are made with a grain, usually rice, and one or two Chinese herbs. Because everything that is eaten must be transformed into 100°—soup before any further digestion and assimilation can begin, soups and porridges are an especially healthful way of eating. When such soups and porridges are made with Chinese herbs as part of their ingredients, then truly, "Medicinals and food have a common source." Below are several Chinese medicinal porridge recipes which can be used for the treatment of rheumatic complaints.

Wu Dou Zhou (Black Bean Congee)

This porridge is made from black soybeans, 30g, white or brown rice, 100g, and a little brown sugar to taste unless one suffers from hypoglycemia or candidiasis and is thus very sensitive to any sugar at all. Soak the black soybeans in water overnight. Then cook the beans and rice into a porridge in one liter of water. Eat once or twice each day. This congee helps expel wind and quicken the blood, disinhibits dampness and disperses swelling. It can be used for wind damp *bi* with swelling, heaviness, and soreness of the joints.

Yi Mi Zhou (Coix Congee)

This porridge only consists of a single ingredient, Semen Coicis Lachryma-jobi (*Yi Yi Ren*). Take 50g of Coix or Job's tears barley and cook with a suitable amount of water to make a thin gruel. As long as one is not overly sensitive to sugar, one may add just a little brown sugar to taste. This congee fortifies the spleen and eliminates dampness and can also be used to treat damp *bi*.

Although Coix does not clear heat, it can be used to treat damp heat *bi* as long as some other treatment is used to help clear the heat.

Cang Er Zi Zhou (Xanthium Seed Congee)

This porridge dispels wind and scatters cold, brightens the eyes, sharpens the hearing, and opens a blocked nose. It can be used to treat wind, cold, damp *bi* as well as headache, stuffy nose, and toothache. It is made from Fructus Xanthii Sibirici (*Cang Er Zi*), 15g and white or brown rice, 50g. First dry fry the Xanthium seeds till they turn yellow. Then boil them in 200ml of water down to 100ml of liquid. Add this liquid to the rice along with another 400ml of water and cook the rice into porridge. Eat this warm two times per day.

Da Ma Zhou (Cannabis Congee)

This porridge is made out of Semen Cannabis Sativae (*Huo Ma Ren*), 10g, and white or brown rice, 50g. First mash the Cannabis seeds and boil them in water. Afterwards, add the resulting liquid to the rice and cook it into a thin gruel. Eat one time each morning and night. This congee moistens the intestines and quickens the blood. It can help treat wind *bi* complicated by blood vacuity dryness. This manifests as constipation, pallor, and inhibition of the joints which are especially stiff.

Ye Jiao Teng Zhou (Polygonum Vine Congee)

This porridge nourishes the blood and quiets the spirit, dispels wind and frees the flow of the network vessels. It can be used to treat restlessness, insomnia, and dream-disturbed sleep but also wind damp *bi* conditions. It is made by cooking 50g of white or brown rice with two Red Dates (Fructus Zizyphi Jujubae, *Da Zao*), and 60g of Caulis Polygoni Multiflori (*Ye Jiao Teng*). First decoct the Polygonum in 500ml of water, remove the dregs, and add the resulting liquid to the rice and Red Dates. Add another 200ml of water and cook into porridge. Eat warm one hour before bed each evening for insomnia. As long as you do not react badly to sugar, you can add a little brown sugar or honey to taste.

For more information on the healing benefits of Chinese medicinal porridges and for even more recipes, see Bob Flaws's *The Book of Jook: Chinese Medicinal Porridges* also published by Blue Poppy Press.

Chinese herbal liniments & plasters

There are a number of different ready-made Chinese plasters to use in the treatment of rheumatic complaints and joint pain. Below is a description of several of these. These may be purchased from Chinese apothecaries in Chinatowns in major American cities and are sometimes available in health food stores or through the mail.

Jing Zhi Gou Pi Gao (Manufactured Essence Dog Skin Plaster, simply called Rheumatic Plaster on the box)

This is one of the very common adhesive plasters manufactured in China for the local topical treatment of rheumatic complaints. Traditionally, an herbal paste was smeared on dog skin in order to make healing poultices. However, nowadays, adhesive backed cotton plasters impregnated with Chinese herbal extracts are used instead. Only the name "dog skin" remains. The ingredients in this popular plaster are meant to aromatically penetrate through the skin and strongly move the qi and quicken the blood. These plasters can be used for any kind of rheumatic or traumatic pain. They are not specific to wind, damp, cold, or heat *bi*.

Apply one plaster over the area of pain and leave in place for 24 hours. A single plaster can also be cut into two or more smaller plasters to cover smaller areas. Do not wear in the bathtub or shower. Do not apply over open wounds or skin lesions. If the plaster causes a blister or other skin irritation, remove it at once.

As long as the area stays irritated, it will actually continue promote healing of the underlying tissues. This is called "counterirritation" and is a very old medical principle used all over the world.

She Xiang Zhui Feng Gao (Musk Expelling Wind Plaster)

This plaster also contains strongly aromatic and penetrating medicinals which move the qi and quicken the blood. Like the plaster above, it is nonspecific for various types of impediment as well as for blood stasis pain. Apply and use the same as above.

Shang Shi Zhi Tong Gao (Damage Due to Dampness, Stop Pain Plaster)

This plaster works the same as the preceding two. Although it contains the word dampness in its name, in fact, it can be used for any type of *bi* or blood stasis due to traumatic injury. Apply and use as above. Another product with a similar name is *Shang Shi Bao Zhen Gao* (Damage Due to Dampness Protect the True Plaster).

Shen Xian Jin Bu Huan Gao (Magic Immortal Not To Be Exchanged for Gold Plaster, also simply called Magic Plaster)

This plaster can be used for wind, cold, damp *bi* or for blood stasis. It consists of a large glob of hardened herbs on a cloth backing. The herbs are mixed with beeswax. To use, one can either steam the plaster until the wax softens or put it in a toaster oven on low to warm it up and melt the wax. When the wax has become soft, apply the plaster to the affected area. However, take care not to apply it too hot or it will cause a nasty burn. If the plaster falls off, one can heat it up a second time and use it again. If the skin becomes irritated or the plaster causes blistering, remove and discontinue its use.

127

Bao Xin An You (Protect the Peace of the Heart Oil, also called *Po Sum On* Medicated Oil)

This medicated oil can be applied topically to the affected joint or body part. It contains similar aromatic, penetrating, qi-moving, and blood-quickening ingredients to the above plasters. It can be used for wind, cold, damp *bi* or blood stasis joint pain and rheumatic complaints. It is often used with either Chinese self-massage or professionally administered Chinese medical massage. Apply directly to the skin liberally and often. Do not get in the eyes. Wash the hands after application, and do not touch the genitalia while this oil is still on the hands. This oil will stain one's clothes, but it can be removed with rubbing alcohol.

All the plasters and liniments discussed above are ready-made and can be purchased from appropriate sources. Below are several recipes for liniments which you can make in your own home.

Shao Lin Wu Xiang Jiu (Shaolin Five Fragrances Wine)

The Shaolin Monastery is famous in Chinese lore for being the home of esoteric martial and healing arts. The following recipe is an authentic one from the Shaolin Monastery. It quickens the blood and scatters stasis, disperses swelling and stops pain. It can be used to treat traumatic injuries as well as wind, damp, cold *bi* conditions. Its ingredients consist of: Flos Caryophylli (*Ding Xiang*), 9g, Radix Auklandiae Lappae (*Mu Xiang*), 9g, Resina Olibani (*Ru Xiang*), 9g, Lignum Santali Albi (*Bai Tan Xiang*), 9g, Fructus Foeniculi Vulgaris (*Xiao Hui Xiang*), 9g, Radix Angelicae Sinensis (*Dang Gui*), 30g, Radix Ligustici Wallichii (*Chuan Xiong*), 24g, Lignum Sappan (*Su Mu*), 24g, Radix Achyranthis Bidentatae (*Niu Xi*), 24g, Flos Carthami Tinctorii (*Hong Hua*), 15g. Place these ingredients in a large lidded pot or jar. Add 500ml of rubbing alcohol and allow to steep for one month, shaking often. After one month, remove the dregs and bottle for use. Apply topically to the affected area several times per day.

Unnamed liniment recipes

1. Take Resina Myrrhae (*Mo Yao*), 3g, Resina Olibani (*Ru Xiang*), 3g, Lacca Sinica Exsiccata (*Shan Qi*), 3g, Flos Carthami Tinctorii (*Hong Hua*), 3g, Borneol (*Bing Pian*), 0.8g, Radix Auklandiae Lappae (*Mu Xiang*), 1g, Camphor (*Zhang Nao*), 6g, Sanguis Draconis (*Xue Jie*), 9g, and soak in one quart of rubbing alcohol for two weeks. Remove the dregs and bottle for use. Apply topically to the affected area for the treatment of blood stasis due to traumatic injury as well as for pain due to wind, cold, damp *bi*.

2. Take 30g each of Flos Carthami Tinctorii (*Hong Hua*), Radix Aconiti (*Chuan Wu*), Radix Aconiti (*Cao Wu*), Extremitas Radicis Angelicae Sinensis (*Gui Wei*), Semen Pruni Persicae (*Tao Ren*), Radix Glycyrrhizae (*Gan Cao*), uncooked Rhizoma Zingiberis (*Sheng Jiang*), Herba Ephedrae (*Ma Huang*), Pyritum (*Zi Ran Tong*), Semen Strychnotis (*Ma Qian Zi*), Ramulus Cinnamomi Cassiae (*Gui Zhi*), Radix Auklandiae Lappae (*Mu Xiang*), and Resina Myrrhae (*Mo Yao*) and put in a large lidded jar or bottle. Add one quart of rubbing alcohol and allow to soak for two weeks. Shake often. Then remove the dregs and bottle for use. Apply topically to the affected area. *Do not use internally!* This liniment is better for wind, cold, damp *bi* and not as good for traumatic injuries as the previous formula.

3. Take Herba Ephedrae (*Ma Huang*), 21g, Ramulus Mori Albi (*Sang Zhi*), 9g, Radix Ledebouriellae Divaricatae (*Fang Feng*), 6g, Zaocys Dhumnades (*Wu Shao She*), 12g, Bombyx Batryticatus (*Tian Chong*), 3g, Flos Carthami Tinctorii (*Hong Hua*), 15g, Radix Aconiti (*Chuan Wu*), 9g, Radix Angelicae Dahuricae (*Bai Zhi*), 6g, Radix Et Rhizoma Notopterygii (*Qiang Huo*), 3g, Radix Angelicae Pubescentis (*Du Huo*), 3g, Cortex Radicis Dictamni Dasycarpi (*Bai Xian Pi*), 6g, Herba Siegesbeckiae (*Xi Xian Cao*), 9g and soak in one quart of rubbing alcohol for two weeks. This liniment is suitable for wind, damp, cold *bi* which is more deep-seated and chronic than the above.

129

Chinese herbal soaks

And finally, it is possible to also treat various painful joints and body parts due to wind, damp, cold *bi* by immersing the affected joint or body part in a hot medicinal soak. One such soak can be made by taking 9g each of Radix Et Rhizoma Notopterygii (*Qiang Huo*), Radix Angelicae Pubescentis (*Du Huo*), Resina Olibani (*Ru Xiang*), Resina Myrrhae (*Mo Yao*), Radix Aconiti (*Chuan Wu*), Radix Aconiti (*Cao Wu*), Herba Lycopodii Cernui (*Shen Jin Cao*), Ramulus Cinnamomi Cassiae (*Gui Zhi*), Fructus Cheanomelis Lagenariae (*Mu Gua*), Fructus Liquidambaris Taiwaniae (*Lu Lu Tong*), Rhizoma Acori Graminei (*Shi Chang Pu*), Eupolyphaga Seu Ophistoplatia (*Tu Bie Chong*), and Flos Carthami Tinctorii (*Hong Hua*). Boil these ingredients in a big pot of water for 15-30 minutes. Remove the dregs and allow to cool to the hottest temperature you can bear without burning yourself. Soak the affected area for 15 minutes. Then be sure to dry and cover the affected area afterwards so that it does not become chilled. This can be done one or two times per day. The same medicinals can be reboiled for several days in a row before changing to fresh ones. This method is especially good for treating either hand or foot *bi*.

All the Chinese medicinals described in the recipes under Chinese medicinal wines, teas, porridges, liniments, and soaks can be purchased through the mail from:

China Herb Co.
165 W. Queen Lane
Philadelphia, PA 19144
Tel: 215-843-5864
Fax: 215-849-3338
Orders: 800-221-4372

When using any Chinese medicinal in any form, if there are any side effects, stop immediately and seek a consultation with a professional practitioner of Chinese medicine.

Learning to live with pain

Not all pain is curable. If joints are too badly damaged or deformed, there is only so much healing that can take place. However, even in such cases, there are a wide range of possibilities that can make living with pain more bearable. There is one in particular that I would like to share and which I have personally seen to be helpful for a number of people with ongoing pain.

The painful sensations in our body ebb and flow. When our attention is continuously focused on the sensation of pain and ridding ourselves of those sensations, our world becomes very small. Our pain becomes the center of the universe with everything revolving around it.

If there is a larger vision and purpose to our life, our suffering is included in that larger field. The sensations of pain may be present, but they are balanced within the larger scope of what we want to accomplish in life. If we have a meaningful mission or goal, the physical sensations of our body may be unpleasant, but they will not stop us from living a full and productive life. The simple fact of the matter is, those who have something to do with their life suffer from pain less than those whose life revolves around their pain and disease.

If you are currently suffering from a rheumatic condition, I wholeheartedly encourage you, for your own sake, to begin working on a life mission statement or a life goal list. Many of us when first hearing this may think that a mission statement is only drawn up by high powered executives like Donald Trump or religious idealists such as Mother Theresa or Ghandi. I have met ordinary people who, after "contracting" RA, refocused their lives through the creation of a mission statement and began to engage in activities that gave new meaning and renewed purpose to their lives. An excellent book that can lead you through the process of developing such a statement is *The Path* by Laurie Beth Jones. As one motivational speaker likes to say "It's not what happens to us, but what we do with it that counts."

Conclusion

The ideas and practices presented in this chapter are like cooking recipes. Just reading a cookbook without actually preparing the recipes can be entertaining, but it will not satisfy your hunger. The same is true for the suggestions offered here. I can tell you these practices have been helpful for thousands of years but that will not satisfy your need, your hunger, unless you see for yourself. Therefore, the practices on these pages need to be put into daily practice. They need to be cooked and baked in your experience. You don't need to do all of them. That is both impossible and unnecessary. Simply find one or two that intrigue you or make sense to try, and begin. Begin today. Nothing of worth is ever been accomplished without some effort.

Finding a Professional Practitioner of Chinese Medicine

Traditional Chinese medicine is one of the fastest growing holistic health care systems in the West today. At the present time, there are 50 colleges in the United States alone which offer three-four year training programs in acupuncture, moxibustion, Chinese herbal medicine, and Chinese medical massage. In addition, many of the graduates of these programs have done postgraduate studies at colleges and hospitals in China, Taiwan, Hong Kong, and Japan. Further, a growing number of trained Oriental medical practitioners have immigrated from China, Japan, and Korea to practice acupuncture and Chinese herbal medicine in the West.

Traditional Chinese medicine, including acupuncture, is a discreet and independent health care profession. It is not simply a technique that can easily be added to the array of techniques of some other health care profession. The study of Chinese medicine, acupuncture, and Chinese herbs is as rigorous as is the study of allopathic, chiropractic, naturopathic, or homeopathic medicine. Previous training in any one of these other systems does not automatically confer competence or knowledge in Chinese medicine. In order to get the full benefits and safety of Chinese medicine, one should seek out professionally trained and credentialed practitioners.

In the United States, recognition that acupuncture and Chinese medicine are their own independent professions has led to the creation of the National Commission for the Certification of Acupuncture & Oriental Medicine (NCCAOM). This commission has created and administers a national board examination in both acupuncture and Chinese herbal medicine in order to insure minimum levels of professional competence and safety. Those who pass the acupuncture exam append the letters Dipl.Ac. (Diplomate of Acupuncture) after their names, while those who pass the Chinese herbal exam use the letters Dipl.C.H. (Diplomate of Chinese Herbs). I recommend that persons wishing to experience the benefits of acupuncture and Chinese medicine should seek treatment in the U.S. only from those who are NCCAOM certified.

In addition, in the United States, acupuncture is a legal, independent health care profession in more than half the states. A few other states require acupuncturists to work under the supervision of MDs, while in a number of states, acupuncture has yet to receive legal status. In states where acupuncture is licensed and regulated, the names of acupuncture practitioners can be found in the *Yellow Pages* of your local phone book or through contacting your State Department of Health, Board of Medical Examiners, or Department of Regulatory Agencies. In states without licensure, it is doubly important to seek treatment only from NCCAOM diplomates.

When seeking a qualified and knowledgeable practitioner, word of mouth referrals are important. Satisfied patients are the most reliable credential a practitioner can have. It is appropriate to ask the practitioner for references from previous patients treated for the same problem. It is best to work with a practitioner who communicates effectively enough for the patient to feel understood and for the Chinese medical diagnosis and treatment plan to make sense. In all cases, a professional practitioner of Chinese medicine should be able and willing to give a written traditional Chinese diagnosis of the patient's pattern upon request.

For further information regarding the practice of Chinese medicine and acupuncture in the United States of America and for referrals to local professional associations and practitioners in the United States, prospective patients may contact:

National Commission for the Certification of Acupuncture & Oriental Medicine
P.O. Box 97075
Washington DC. 20090-7075
Tel: (202) 232-1404
Fax: (202) 462-6157

The National Acupuncture & Oriental Medicine Alliance
14637 Starr Rd, SE
Olalla, WA 98357
Tel: (206) 851-6895
Fax: (206) 728-4841
E mail: 76143.2061@compuserve.com

The American Association of Oriental Medicine
433 Front St.
Catasauqua, PA 18032-2506
Tel: (610) 433-2448
Fax: (610) 433-1832

Learning More About Chinese Medicine

For more information on Chinese medicine in general, see:

The Web That Has No Weaver: Understanding Chinese Medicine by Ted Kaptchuk, Congdon & Weed, NY, 1983. This is the best overall introduction to Chinese medicine for the serious lay reader. It has been a standard since it was first published over a dozen years ago and it has yet to be replaced.

Chinese Secrets of Health & Longevity by Bob Flaws, Sound True, Boulder, CO, 1996. This is a six tape audio cassette course introducing Chinese medicine to laypeople. It covers basic Chinese medical theory, Chinese dietary therapy, Chinese herbal medicine, acupuncture, *qi gong*, *feng shui*, deep relaxation, lifestyle, and more.

Fundamentals of Chinese Medicine by the East Asian Medical Studies Society, Paradigm Publications, Brookline, MA, 1985. This is a more technical introduction and overview of Chinese medicine intended for professional entry level students.

Traditional Medicine in Contemporary China by Nathan Sivin, Center for Chinese Studies, University of Michigan, Ann Arbor, 1987. This book discusses the development of Chinese medicine in China in the last half century.

Imperial Secrets of Health and Longevity by Bob Flaws, Blue Poppy Press, Boulder, CO, 1994. This book includes a section on Chinese dietary therapy and generally introduces the basic concepts of good health according to Chinese medicine.

Chinese Herbal Remedies by Albert Y. Leung, Universe Books, NY, 1984. This book is about simple Chinese herbal home remedies.

Legendary Chinese Healing Herbs by Henry C. Lu, Sterling Publishing, Inc., NY, 1991. This book is a fun way to begin learning about Chinese herbal medicine. It is full of interesting and entertaining anecdotes about Chinese medicinal herbs.

The Mystery of Longevity by Liu Zheng-cai, Foreign Languages Press, Beijing, 1990. This book is also about general principles and practice promoting good health according to Chinese medicine.

For more information on Chinese rheumatology, see:

Bi-Syndromes or Rheumatic Disorders Treated by Traditional Chinese Medicine by L. Vangermeersch & Sun Pei-lin, SATAS, Belgium, 1994. This is a professional level clinical manual on *bi* conditions in Chinese medicine. It discusses the Chinese theory of rheumatic complaints and gives both acupuncture and Chinese medicinal treatments. Included is a nice *materia medica* of the commonly used Chinese herbs for *bi* conditions. There are also a number of charts showing the locations of acupuncture points commonly used in treating rheumatic complaints.

Rheumatology in Chinese Medicine by Gérard Guillaume & Mach Chieu, Eastland Press, Seattle, 1996. This is an even bigger, more complete professional level discussion of rheumatology in Chinese medicine. Its emphasis is more on acupuncture than on herbal medicine.

138

For more information on Chinese dietary therapy, see:

The Dao of Healthy Eating According to Chinese Medicine by Bob Flaws, Blue Poppy Press, Boulder, CO, 1997. This book is a layperson's primer on Chinese dietary therapy. It includes detailed sections on the clear, bland diet as well as sections on chronic candidiasis and allergies, as well as specifics of food energetics.

Prince Wen Hui's Cook: Chinese Dietary Therapy by Bob Flaws & Honora Lee Wolfe, Paradigm Publications, Brookline, MA, 1983. This book is an introduction to Chinese dietary therapy. Although some of the information it contains is dated, it does give the Chinese medicinal descriptions of most foods commonly eaten in the West.

The Book of Jook: Chinese Medicinal Porridges, a Healthy Alternative to the Typical Western Breakfast by Bob Flaws, Blue Poppy Press, Boulder, CO, 1995. This book is specifically about Chinese medicinal porridges made with very simple combinations of Chinese medicinal herbs.

Chinese Medicinal Wines & Elixirs by Bob Flaws, Blue Poppy Press, Boulder, CO, 1995. This book is a large collection of simple, one, two, and three ingredient Chinese medicinal wines which can be made at home.

Chinese Medicinal Teas: Simple, Proven Folk Formulas for Common Diseases & Promoting Health by Zong Xiao-fan & Gary Liscum, Blue Poppy Press, Boulder, CO, 1997. Like the above two books, this book is about one, two, and three ingredient Chinese medicinal teas which are easy to make and can be used at home as adjuncts to other, professionally prescribed treatments or for the promotion of health and prevention of disease.

The Tao of Nutrition by Maoshing Ni, Union of Tao and Man, Los Angeles, 1989

Harmony Rules: The Chinese Way of Health Through Food by Gary Butt & Frena Bloomfield, Samuel Weiser, Inc., York Beach, ME, 1985

Chinese System of Food Cures: Prevention & Remedies by Henry C. Lu, Sterling Publishing Co., Inc, NY, 1986

A Practical English-Chinese Library of Traditional Chinese Medicine: Chinese Medicated Diet ed. by Zhang En-qin, Shanghai College of Traditional Chinese Medicine Publishing House, Shanghai, 1990

Eating Your Way to Health — Dietotherapy in Traditional Chinese Medicine by Cai Jing-feng, Foreign Languages Press, Beijing, 1988

For more information on *qi gong*, see:

Chi Kung: Cultivating Personal Energy by James MacRitchie, Element, Shaftesbury, UK, 1993. This is a short, well-written introduction to *qi gong*. It includes the history and theory of *qi gong* as well as a selection of different *qi gong* exercises.

The Chinese Exercise Book by Dahong Zhou, Hartley & Marks, Pt. Roberts, WA, 1984. This book teaches several of the most famous systems of *qi gong*. In addition, it has special sections for the elderly and *qi gong* for particular diseases, including sciatica and lumbar disk problems.

Exercises Illustrated: Ancient Way to Keep Fit by Zong Wu & Li Mao, Shelter Publications, Inc., Bolinas, CA, 1992. This is a very beautiful book filled with ancient and modern Chinese drawings and painting of various *qi gong* exercises.

Qigong for Arthritis by Yang Jing-ming, Yang's Martial Arts Association, Jamaica Plain, NY, 1991. This book focuses on the healing benefits of *qi gong* specifically for arthritis.

Change the Picture: A Qigong Workbook by Yu-cheng Huang, Ching Ying Tai Chi Kung Fu Association, Chicago, IL. This book presents a systematic, progressive regimen for learning *qi gong*. Theory and method are provided in a series of self-study lessons allowing the student to increase their understanding and ability with *qi gong* through practice of a series of well-illustrated exercises designed to learn to feel the qi, lead the qi, supplement the qi, etc.

Knocking At the Gate of Life by Edward C. Chang, Rodale Press Inc., Emmaus, PA. This book presents *qi gong* exercises for hundreds of different health problems.

Qigong / Chi Kung: Awakening and Mastering the Medicine Within You by Roger Jahnke, Health Action, Santa Barbara, CA, undated. This is an excellent videotape for learning to do *qi gong*. A number of very simple yet effective exercises are given designed to improve health and treat disease.

Qigong: The Chinese Way of Health by Ken Cohen, Nederland, CO. This one hour videotape covers the two most basic form of *qi gong*, the Six Healing Sounds and Standing Meditation. In particular, the Six Healing Sounds are useful for treating disease due to dysfunction of the internal organs.

The Way of Qigong: The Art and Science of Chinese Energy Healing by Kenneth S. Cohen, Ballantine Books, NY, 1997. This book is, in my opinion, the single best book on *qi gong*. Although perhaps a little scholarly for some people's taste, this book presents the history of *qi gong*, explains the different types of *qi gong*, and includes basic guidelines for safe and effective *qi gong* practice.

141

Chinese Medical Glossary

C hinese medicine is a system unto itself. Its technical terms are uniquely its own and cannot be reduced to the definitions of Western medicine without destroying the very fabric and logic of Chinese medicine. Ultimately, because Chinese medicine was created in the Chinese language, Chinese medicine is best and really only understood in that language. Nevertheless, as Westerners trying to understand Chinese medicine, we must translate the technical terms of Chinese medicine into English words. If some of these technical translations sound at first peculiar and their meaning is not immediately transparent, this is because no equivalent concepts exist in everyday English.

In the past, some Western authors have erroneously translated technical Chinese medical terms using Western medical or at least quasi-scientific words in an attempt to make this system more acceptable to Western audiences. For instance, the words tonify and sedate are commonly seen in the Western Chinese medical literature even though, in the case of sedate, it meaning is 180° opposite to the Chinese understanding of the word *xie*. *Xie* means to drain off something which has pooled and accumulated. That accumulation is seen as something excess which should not be lingering where it is. Because it is accumulating somewhere where it shouldn't, it is impeding and obstructing whatever should be moving to and through that area. The word sedate comes from the Latin word *sedere*, to sit. Therefore, the word sedate means to make something sit still. In English, we get the word sediment from this same root. However, the Chinese *xie* means draining off which is sitting somewhere erroneously. Therefore, to think that one is going to sedate what is already sitting is a great mistake in understanding the clinical implication and application of this technical term.

Therefore, in order to preserve the integrity of this system while still making it intelligible to English language readers, I have appended the following glossary of Chinese medical technical terms. The terms themselves are based on Nigel Wiseman's *English-Chinese Chinese-English Dictionary of Chinese Medicine* published by the Hunan Science & Technology Press in Changsha, Hunan, People's Republic of China in 1995. Dr. Wiseman is, I believe, the greatest Western scholar in terms of the translation of Chinese medicine into English. As a Chinese reader myself, although I often find Wiseman's terms awkward sounding at first, I also think they convey most accurately the Chinese understanding and logic of these terms.

Vacuity: Emptiness or insufficiency, typically of qi, blood, yin, or yang

Viscera: The solid yin organs of Chinese medicine

Bowels: The hollow yang organs of Chinese medicine

Repletion: Excess or fullness, almost always pathological

Supplement: To add to or augment, as in supplementing the qi, blood, yin, or yang

Drain: To drain off or away some pathological qi or substance from where it is replete or excess

Depression: Stagnation and lack of movement, as in liver depression qi stagnation

Stagnation: Nonmovement of the qi, lack of free flow, constraint

Yin: In the body, substance and nourishment

Yang: In the body, function, movement, activity, transformation

Dampness: A pathological accumulation of body fluids

Phlegm: A pathological accumulation of phlegm or mucus congealed from dampness or body fluids

Qi: Activity, function, that which moves, transforms, defends, restrains, and warms

Blood: The red colored fluids which flow in the vessels and nourishes and constructs the tissues of the body

Channels: The main routes for the distribution of qi and blood, but mainly qi

Vessels: The main routes for the distribution of qi and blood, but mainly blood

Network vessels: Small vessels which form a net-like web insuring the flow of qi and blood to all body tissues

Counterflow: An erroneous flow of qi, usually upward but sometimes horizontally as well

Spirit: The accumulation of qi in the heart which manifests as consciousness, sensory awareness, and mental-emotional function

Essence: A stored, very potent form of substance and qi, usually yin when compared to yang qi, but can be transformed into yang qi

Acquired essence: Essence manufactured out of the surplus of qi and blood in turn created out of the refined essence of food and drink

Acupuncture: The regulation of qi flow by the stimulation of certain points located on the channels and network vessels achieved mainly by insertion of fine needles into these points

Moxibustion: Burning the herb Artemisia Argyium on, over, or near acupuncture points in order to add yang qi, warm cold, or promote the movement of the qi and blood

Hydrotherapy: Using various baths and water applications to treat and prevent disease

Magnet therapy: Applying magnets to acupuncture points to treat and prevent disease

Decoction: A method of administering Chinese medicinals by boiling these medicinals in water, removing the dregs, and drinking the resulting medicinal liquid

Qi mechanism: The process of transforming yin substance controlled and promoted by the qi, largely synonymous with the process of digestion

Clear: The pure or clear part of food and drink ingested which is then turned into qi and blood

Turbid: The yin, impure, turbid part of food and drink which is sent downward to be excreted as waste

145

Acupoints: Those places on the channels and network vessels where qi and blood tend to collect in denser concentrations, and thus those places where the qi and blood in the channels are especially available for manipulation

Seven star hammer: A small hammer with needles embedded in its head used to stimulate acupoints without actually inserting needles

Qi vacuity: Insufficient qi manifesting in diminished movement, transformation, and function

Blood vacuity: Insufficient blood manifesting in diminished nourishment, construction, and moistening of body tissues

Yin vacuity: Insufficient yin substance necessary to both nourish, control, and counterbalance yang activity

Vacuity heat: Heat due to hyperactive yang in turn due to insufficient controlling yin

Yang vacuity: Insufficient warming and transforming function giving rise to symptoms of cold in the body

Life gate fire: Another name for kidney yang or kidney fire, seen as the ultimate source of yang qi in the body

Blood stasis: Also called dead blood, malign blood, and dry blood, blood stasis is blood which is no longer moving through the vessels as it should. Instead it is precipitated in the vessels like silt in a river. Like silt, it then obstructs the free flow of the blood in the vessels and also impedes the production of new or fresh blood.

Portals: Also called orifices, the openings of the sensory organs and the opening of the heart through which the spirit makes contact with the world outside

Five phase theory: An ancient Chinese system of correspondences dividing up all of reality into five phases which then mutually engender and check each other according to definite sequences

Heat toxins: A particularly virulent and concentrated type of pathological heat often associated with purulence (*i.e.*, pus formation), sores, and sometimes, but not always, malignancies

Depressive heat: Heat due to enduring or severe qi stagnation which then transforms into heat

Damp heat: A combination of accumulated dampness mixed with pathological heat often associated with sores, abnormal vaginal discharges, and some types of menstrual and body pain

Lassitude of the spirit: A listless of apathetic affect or emotional demeanor due to obvious fatigue of the mind and body

Bedroom taxation: Fatigue or vacuity due to excessive sex

Central qi: Also called the middle qi, this is synonymous with the spleen-stomach qi

Vacuity cold: Obvious signs and symptoms of cold due to a lack or insufficiency of yang qi

Impediment: A hindrance to the free flow of the qi and blood typically manifesting as pain and restriction in the range of movement of a joint or extremity

Environmental excesses: A superabundance of wind, cold, dampness, dryness, heat, or summerheat in the external environment which can invade the body and cause disease

External causes of disease: The six environmental excesses

Internal causes of disease: The seven affects or emotions, namely, anger, joy (or excitement), sorrow, thought, fear, melancholy, and fright

Neither external nor internal causes of disease: a miscellaneous group of pathogenic factors including trauma, diet, overtaxation, insufficient exercise, poisoning, parasites, etc.

Defensive qi: The yang qi which protects the exterior of the body from invasion by the environmental excesses

Constructive qi: The qi which flows through the channels and nourishes and constructs the internal organs and body tissues

Bibliography

Chinese language sources

Cheng Dan An Zhen Jiu Xuan Ji (Cheng Dan-an's Selected Acupuncture & Moxibustion Works), ed. by Cheng Wei-fen *et al.*, Shanghai Science & Technology Press, Shanghai, 1986

Chu Zhen Zhi Liao Xue (A Study of Acupuncture Treatment), Li Zhong-yu, Sichuan Science & Technology Press, Chengdu, 1990

Dong Yuan Yi Ji (Dong-yuan's Collected Medical Works), ed. by Bao Zheng-fei *et al.*, People's Health & Hygiene Press, Beijing, 1993

Han Ying Chang Yong Yi Xue Ci Hui (Chinese-English Glossary of Commonly Used Medical Terms), Huang Xiao-kai, Peoples Health & Hygeine Press, Beijing, 1982

Shang Hai Lao Zhong Yi Jing Yan Xuan Bian (A Selected Compilation of Shanghai Old Doctors' Experiences), Shanghai Science & Technology Press, Shanghai, 1984

Shi Yong Zhen Jiu Tui Na Zhi Liao Xue (A Study of Practical Acupuncture, Moxibustion & Tui Na Treatments), Xia Zhi-ping, Shanghai College of Chinese Medicine Press, Shanghai, 1990

Tan Zheng Lun (Treatise on Phlegm Conditions), Hou Tian-yin & Wang Chun-hua, People's Army Press, Beijing, 1989

Yi Zong Jin Jian (The Golden Mirror of Ancestral Medicine), Wu Qian *et al.*, People's Health & Hygeine Press, Beijing, 1985

Yu Xue Zheng Zhi (Static Blood Patterns & Treatments), Zhang Xue-wen, Shanxi Science & Technology Press, Xian, 1986

Zhen Jiu Da Cheng (A Great Compendium of Acupuncture & Moxibustion), Yang Ji-zhou, People's Health & Hygiene Press, Beijing, 1983

Zhen Jiu Xue (A Study of Acupuncture & Moxibustion), Qiu Mao-liang *et al.*, Shanghai Science & Technology Press, Shanghai, 1985

Zhen Jiu Yi Xue (An Easy Study of Acupuncture & Moxibustion), Li Shou-xian, People's Health & Hygiene Press, Beijing, 1990

Zhong Guo Min Jian Cao Yao Fang (Chinese Folk Herbal Medicinal Formulas), Liu Guang-rui & Liu Shao-lin, Sichuan Science & Technology Press, Chengdu, 1992

Zhong Guo Zhen Jiu Chu Fang Xue (A Study of Chinese Acupuncture & Moxibustion Prescriptions), Xiao Shao-qing, Ningxia People's Press, Yinchuan, 1986

Zhong Guo Zhong Yi Mi Fang Da Quan (A Great Compendium of Chinese National Chinese Medical Secret Formulas), ed. by Hu Zhao-ming, Literary Propagation Publishing Company, Shanghai, 1992

Zhong Yi Hu Li Xue (A Study of Chinese Medical Nursing), Lu Su-ying, People's Health & Hygiene Press, Beijing, 1983

Zhong Yi Lin Chuang Ge Ke (Various Clinical Specialties in Chinese Medicine), Zhang En-qin *et al.*, Shanghai College of TCM Press, Shanghai, 1990

Zhong Yi Ling Yan Fang (Efficacious Chinese Medical Formulas), Lin Bin-zhi, Science & Technology Propagation Press, Beijing, 1991

English language sources

A Barefoot Doctor's Manual, revised & enlarged edition, Cloudburst Press, Mayne Isle, 1977

A Clinical Guide to Chinese Herbs and Formulae, Cheng Song-yu & Li Fei, Churchill & Livingstone, Edinburgh, 1993

A Compendium of TCM Patterns & Treatments, Bob Flaws & Daniel Finney, Blue Poppy Press, Boulder, CO, 1996

A Comprehensive Guide to Chinese Herbal Medicine, Chen Ze-lin & Chen Mei-fang, Oriental Healing Arts Institute, Long Beach, CA, 1992

All About Arthritis, Derrick Brewerton, Harvard University Press, Cambridge, MA, 1992

The Dao of Healthy Eating According to Chinese Medicine, Bob Flaws, Blue Poppy Press, Boulder, CO, 1997

"Aspirin and Bleeding Peptic Ulcers in the Elderly", G. Faulkner *et al.*, *British Medical Journal*, 1988:297:1311-13

A Handbook of Differential Diagnosis with Key Signs & Symptoms, Therapeutic Principles, and Guiding Prescriptions, Ouyang Yi, trans. by C. S. Cheung, Harmonious Sunshine Cultural Center, San Francisco, 1987

Between Heaven and Earth, Harriet Beinfeld & Efrem Korngold, Ballantine Books, NY, 1991

Bi-Syndromes or Rheumatic Disorders Treated by Traditional Chinese Medicine, L. Vangermeersch & Sun Pei-lin, SATAS, Belgium, 1994

Candida and Candidosis, F. C. Odds, University Park Press, Baltimore, 1979

Chinese-English Terminology of Traditional Chinese Medicine, Shuai Xue-zhong *et al.*, Hunan Science & Technology Press, Changsha, 1983

Chinese-English Manual of Common-used Prescriptions in Traditional Chinese Medicine, ed. by Ou Ming, Joint Publishing Co., Ltd., Hong Kong, 1989

Chinese Herbal Medicine: Formulas & Strategies, Dan Bensky & Randall Barolet, Eastland Press, Seattle, 1990

Chinese Herbal Medicine: Materia Medica, Dan Bensky & Andrew Gamble, second, revised edition, Eastland Press, Seattle, 1993

Chinese Herbal Teas: Simple, Proven Folk Formulas for Common Diseases and Promoting Health, Zong Xiao-fan & Gary Liscum, Blue Poppy Press, Boulder, CO, 1997

Chinese Medicinal Wines & Elixirs, Bob Flaws, Blue Poppy Press, Boulder, CO, 1995

Chinese Self-massage, The Easy Way to Health, Fan Ya-li, Blue Poppy Press, Boulder, CO, 1996

"Controlled Trial of Fasting and One-year Vegetarian Diet in Rheumatoid Arthritis", Kragh J. Kjeldsen *et al.*, *The Lancet*, 1991; 338:899-902

"Detection of Chlamydia Trachomatis DNA in Joints of Reactive Arthritis Patients by Polymerase Chain Reaction", D. Gilroy Taylor-Robinson, *The Lancet*, 1992;340:81-82

"Diet for Rheumatoid Arthritis", L. G. Darlington & N. W. Ramsey, *The Lancet*, 1991; 338 (8775):1209

"Drug-induced End Stage Renal Disease", P. Ronco & A. Flahault, *New England Journal of Medicine*, Vol. 331, #25, 1994, pp. 1711-12

English-Chinese Chinese-English Dictionary of Chinese Medicine, Nigel Wiseman, Hunan Science & Technology Press, Changsha, 1995

"Epidemiology of Adverse Reactions to Nonsteroidal Anti-inflammatory Drugs", J.C.P. Weber, *Advances in Inflammation*, Raven Press, NY, 1984

"Fasting and Vegan Diet in Rheumatoid Arthritis", L. Skoldstam, *Scandinavian Journal of Rheumatology*, 1986;15:219-23

"Food Allergy or Enterometabolic Disorder?", J.O. Hunter, *The Lancet*, 1991;338:495-96

Fundamentals of Chinese Acupuncture, Andrew Ellis, Nigel Wiseman & Ken Boss, Paradigm Publications, Brookline, MA, 1988

Fundamentals of Chinese Medicine, Nigel Wiseman & Andrew Ellis, Paradigm Publications, Brookline, MA, 1985

Glossary of Chinese Medical Terms and Acupuncture Points, Nigel Wiseman & Ken Boss, Paradigm Publications, Brookline, MA, 1990

Handbook of Chinese Herbs and Formulas, Him-che Yeung, self-published, LA, 1985

"Hepatotoxicity on Nonsteroidal Anti-inflammatory Drugs", R. Mordechai *et al.*, *The American Journal of Gastroenterology*, 1992;87 (12):1696-1704

153

"NSAIDs and Osteoarthritis", P.M. Brooks *et al.*, *Journal of Rheumatology*, 1982; 9:3-5

Oriental Materia Medica, a Concise Guide, Hong-yen Hsu, Oriental Healing Arts Institute, Long Beach, CA, 1986

Practical Traditional Chinese Medicine & Pharmacology: Clinical Experiences, Shang Xian-min *et al.*, New World Press, Beijing, 1990

Practical Traditional Chinese Medicine & Pharmacology: Herbal Formulas, Geng Jun-ying, *et al.*, New World Press, Beijing, 1991

"Prednisone Use in RA", Carol Potera, *Arthritis Today*, March-April, 1995, p. 8

Rheumatology in Chinese Medicine, Gérard Guillaume & Mach Chieu, Eastland Press, Seattle, 1996

Statements of Fact in Traditional Chinese Medicine, Bob Flaws, Blue Poppy Press, Boulder, CO

The Book of Jook: Chinese Medicinal Porridges, Bob Flaws, Blue Poppy Press, Boulder, CO, 1995

The Complete Book of Chinese Health and Healing, Daniel Reid, Shambhala, Boston, 1994

The English-Chinese Encyclopedia of Practical Traditional Chinese Medicine, Xuan Jia-sheng, ed., Higher Education Press, Beijing, 1990

The Essential Book of Traditional Chinese Medicine, Liu Yan-chi, trans. by Fang Ting-yu & Chen Lai-di, Columbia University Press, NY, 1988

The History of Crime Against the Food Law: The Amazing Story of the National Food and Drug Law Intended to Protect the Health of the People Perverted to Protect Adulteration of Foods and Drugs, Harvey W. Wiley, self-published, Washington DC, 1929

The Merck Manual, 15th edition, ed. by Robert Berkow, Merck Sharp & Dohme Research Laboratories, Rahway, NJ, 1987

The Path, Laurie Beth Jones, Hyperion, NY

The Treatise on the Spleen & Stomach, Li Dong-yuan, trans. by Yang Shou-zhong, Blue Poppy Press, Boulder, CO, 1993

The Yeast Connection, William G. Crook, Vintage Books, Random House, NY, 1986

The Yeast Syndrome, John Parks Towbridge & Morton Walker, Bantam Books, Toronto, 1988

Traditional Medicine in Contemporary China, Nathan Sivin, University of Michigan, Ann Arbor, 1987

Zang Fu: The Organ Systems of Traditional Chinese Medicine, second edition, Jeremy Ross, Churchill Livingstone, Edinburgh, 1985

Index

159

Qigong for Arthritis 101, 141

R

relaxation, deep 18, 75, 92-97, 137
relaxation tapes 93, 94
rheumatic *bi* 7, 8, 10, 14-20, 25, 27,
    29, 33, 41, 42, 44, 47, 48, 51, 52,
    58, 60, 61, 63, 64, 67, 71, 78, 89,
    92, 101, 105, 110, 119, 122
rheumatic pain, chronic 59
rheumatic pain, early stage 55
rheumatoid arthritis 2, 4, 5, 41, 60,
    68, 69, 72, 73

S

Salvia & Eucommia Wine 121
San She Dan Zhui Feng Wan 117
seven star hammer 106, 107, 146
Shang Shi Zhi Tong Gao 61, 127
Shao Lin Wu Xiang Jiu 128
Shaolin Five Fragrances Wine 128
Shaolin Monastery 128
She Xiang Zhui Feng Gao 127
Shen Ling Bai Zhu Pian 67
Shen Xian Jin Bu Huan Gao 127
Si Wu Tang 70
Sivin, Nathan 137, 155
small intestine 13
Small Quicken the Network Vessels
    Elixir 64, 117
Specially Effective Low Back Remedy
    117
spleen vacuity 38, 39, 61, 64, 67, 79,
    80, 83, 84, 88, 90
State Department of Health 134
stomach 11, 13, 16, 17, 24, 28, 77, 80,
    86, 111, 123, 147, 155
Sun Pei-lin 138, 151

T

Te Xiao Yao Tong Ling 117
Temple of Heaven Balm 109
The Book of Jook 126, 139, 154
The Merck Manual 1, 4, 155
The Path 96, 131, 155

Theodosakis, Jason 4
thread moxibustion 108, 110
Three Free Therapies 75, 89, 92
Three Snake Gallbladder Expel Wind
    Pills 117
Tian Qi Du Zhong Wan 118
Tiger Balm 109
triple burner 13
tui na 52, 53, 149
Tylenol 4, 5

U, V, W

Unschuld, Paul 9
urinary bladder 13
Vangermeersch, L. 138, 151
vegetarianism 86
viscera & bowels 13
wind 27-30, 33, 37, 41, 42, 51, 55-64,
    67, 71, 100, 105, 107, 109, 113-117,
    119-130, 147
wind damp exterior pattern 55
wind damp heat exterior pattern 57
Wind Damp Tablets 116
wind dampness 33, 116, 117
Wind Dampness Dispersing Pain
    Pills 116
wind, cold, damp bi 59, 61-63, 115,
    116, 122, 125, 127-129
Wiseman, Nigel 153
Wolfe, Honora Lee 139
Wu Dou Zhou 124

X, Y, Z

Xanthium Seed Congee 125
Xiang Sha Liu Jun Zi Tang 64
Xiao Huo Luo Dan 64, 117
Yang Jing-ming 141
Ye Jiao Teng Zhou 125
Yellow Pages 134
Yi Mi Fang Feng Cha 123
Yi Mi Zhou 124
yin & yang 8
Zhang En-qin 140, 150
Zong Wu 140
Zong Xiao-fan 123, 139, 152

OTHER BOOKS ON CHINESE MEDICINE
AVAILABLE FROM BLUE POPPY PRESS

1775 Linden Ave, Boulder, CO 80304
For ordering 1-800-487-9296 PH. 303\447-8372 FAX 303\447-0740

A NEW AMERICAN ACUPUNC-TURE by Mark Seem, ISBN 0-936185-44-9

ACUPUNCTURE AND MOXI-BUSTION FORMULAS & TREAT-MENTS by Cheng Dan-an, trans. by Wu Ming, ISBN 0-936185-68-6

ACUTE ABDOMINAL SYN-DROMES: Their Diagnosis & Treatment by Combined Chinese-Western Medicine by Alon Marcus, ISBN 0-936185-31-7

AGING & BLOOD STASIS: A New Approach to TCM Geriatrics by Yan De-xin, ISBN 0-936185-63-5

AIDS & ITS TREATMENT ACCORDING TO TRADITIONAL CHINESE MEDICINE by Huang Bing-shan, trans. by Fu-Di & Bob Flaws, ISBN 0-936185-28-7

THE BOOK OF JOOK: Chinese Medicinal Porridges, An Alternative to the Typical Western Breakfast by B. Flaws, ISBN0-936185-60-0

CHINESE MEDICAL PALMIS-TRY: Your Health in Your Hand by Zong Xiao-fan & Gary Liscum, ISBN 0-936185-64-3

CHINESE MEDICINAL TEAS: Simple, Proven, Folk Formulas for Common Diseases & Promoting Health by Zong Xiao-fan & Gary Liscum, ISBN 0-936185-76-7

CHINESE MEDICINAL WINES & ELIXIRS by Bob Flaws, ISBN 0-936185-58-9

CHINESE PEDIATRIC MAS-SAGE THERAPY: *A Parent's & Practitioner's Guide to the Prevention & Treatment of Childhood Illness* by Fan Ya-li, ISBN 0-936185-54-6

CHINESE SELF-MASSAGE THE-RAPY: The Easy Way to Health by Fan Ya-li ISBN 0-936185-74-0

CLASSICAL MOXIBUSTION SKILLS in Clinical Practice by Sung Baek, ISBN 0-936185-16-3

A COMPENDIUM OF TCM PAT-TERNS & TREATMENTS by Bob Flaws & Daniel Finney, ISBN 0-936185-70-8

CURING ARTHRITIS NATURALLY WITH CHINESE MEDICINE by Doug Frank & Bob Flaws ISBN 0-936185-87-2

CURING INSOMNIA NATURALLY WITH CHINESE MEDICINE by Bob Flaws ISBN 0-936185-85-6

THE DAO OF INCREASING LONGEVITY AND CONSER-VING ONE'S LIFE by Anna Lin & Bob Flaws, ISBN 0-936185-24-4

THE DAO OF HEALTHY EATING ACCORDING TO CHINESE MEDICINE by Bob Flaws, ISBN 0-936185-92-9

THE DIVINELY RESPONDING CLASSIC: *A Translation of the Shen Ying Jing from Zhen Jiu Da Cheng,* trans. by Yang Shou-zhong & Liu Feng-ting ISBN 0-936185-55-4

DUI YAO: THE ART OF COMBINING CHINESE HERBAL MEDICINALS by Philippe Sionneau ISBN 0-936185-81-3

ENDOMETRIOSIS, INFERTILITY AND TRADITIONAL CHINESE MEDICINE: A Laywoman's Guide by Bob Flaws ISBN 0-936185-14-7

EXTRA TREATISES BASED ON INVESTIGATION & INQUIRY: A Translation of Zhu Dan-xi's Ge Zhi Yu Lun, by Yang Shou-zhong & Duan Wu-jin, ISBN 0-936185-53-8

FIRE IN THE VALLEY: TCM Diagnosis & Treatment of Vaginal Diseases ISBN 0-936185-25-2

FLESHING OUT THE BONES: The Importance of Case Histories in Chin. Med. trans. by Chip Chace. ISBN 0-936185-30-9

FU QING-ZHU'S GYNECOLOGY trans. by Yang Shou-zhong and Liu Da-wei, ISBN 0-936185-35-X

FULFILLING THE ESSENCE: A Handbook of Traditional & Contemporary Treatments for Female Infertility by Bob Flaws, ISBN 0-936185-48-1

GOLDEN NEEDLE WANG LE-TING: A 20th Century Master's Approach to Acupuncture by Yu Hui-chan and Han Fu-ru, trans. by Shuai Xue-zhong,

A HANDBOOK OF TRADITIONAL CHINESE DERMATOLOGY by Liang Jian-hui, trans. by Zhang & Flaws, ISBN 0-936185-07-4

A HANDBOOK OF TRADITIONAL CHINESE GYNECOLOGY by Zhejiang College of TCM, trans. by Zhang Ting-liang, ISBN 0-936185-06-6 (4th edit.)

A HANDBOOK OF MENSTRUAL DISEASES IN CHINESE MEDI-

CINE by Bob Flaws ISBN 0-936185-82-1

A HANDBOOK of TCM PEDIATRICS by Bob Flaws, ISBN 0-936185-72-4

A HANDBOOK OF TCM UROLOGY & MALE SEXUAL DYSFUNCTION by Anna Lin, OMD, ISBN 0-936185-36-8

THE HEART & ESSENCE OF DAN-XI'S METHODS OF TREATMENT by Xu Dan-xi, trans. by Yang, ISBN 0-926185-49-X

THE HEART TRANSMISSION OF MEDICINE by Liu Yi-ren, trans. by Yang Shou-zhong ISBN 0-936185-83-X

HIGHLIGHTS OF ANCIENT ACUPUNCTURE PRESCRIPTIONS trans. by Wolfe & Crescenz ISBN 0-936185-23-6

How to Have A HEALTHY PREGNANCY, HEALTHY BIRTH with Chinese Medicine by Honora Lee Wolfe, ISBN 0-936185-40-6

HOW TO WRITE A TCM HERBAL FORMULA: A Logical Methodology for the Formulation & Administration of Chinese Herbal Medicine in Decoction by Bob Flaws, ISBN 0-936185-49-X

IMPERIAL SECRETS OF HEALTH & LONGEVITY by Bob Flaws, ISBN 0-936185-51-1

KEEPING YOUR CHILD HEALTHY WITH CHINESE MEDICINE by Bob Flaws, ISBN 0-936185-71-6

Li Dong-yuan's TREATISE ON THE SPLEEN & STOMACH, A Translation of the Pi Wei Lun by Yang Shou-zhong & Li Jian-yong, ISBN 0-936185-41-4

LOW BACK PAIN: Care & Prevention with Chinese Medicine by Douglas Frank, ISBN 0-936185-66-X